# 2022

This
Planner
belongs to:

..............................................................................................................

..............................................................................................................

..............................................................................................................

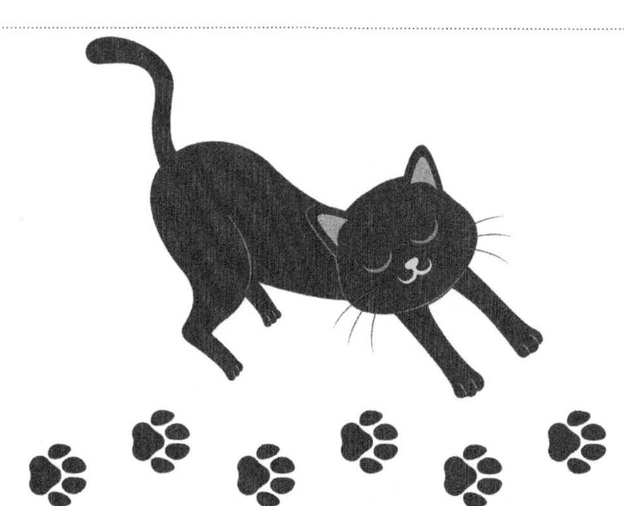

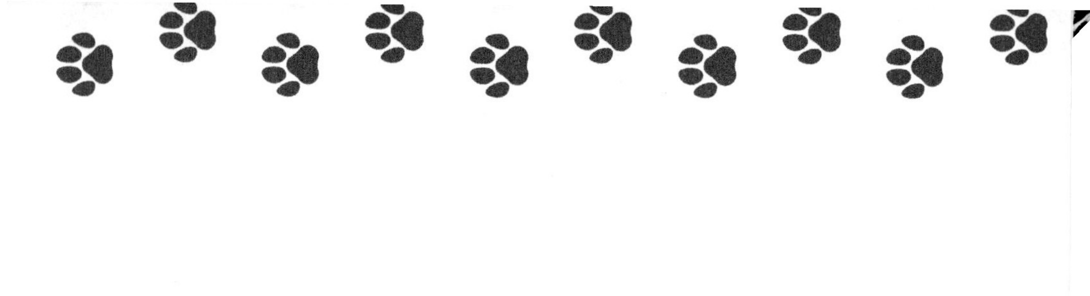

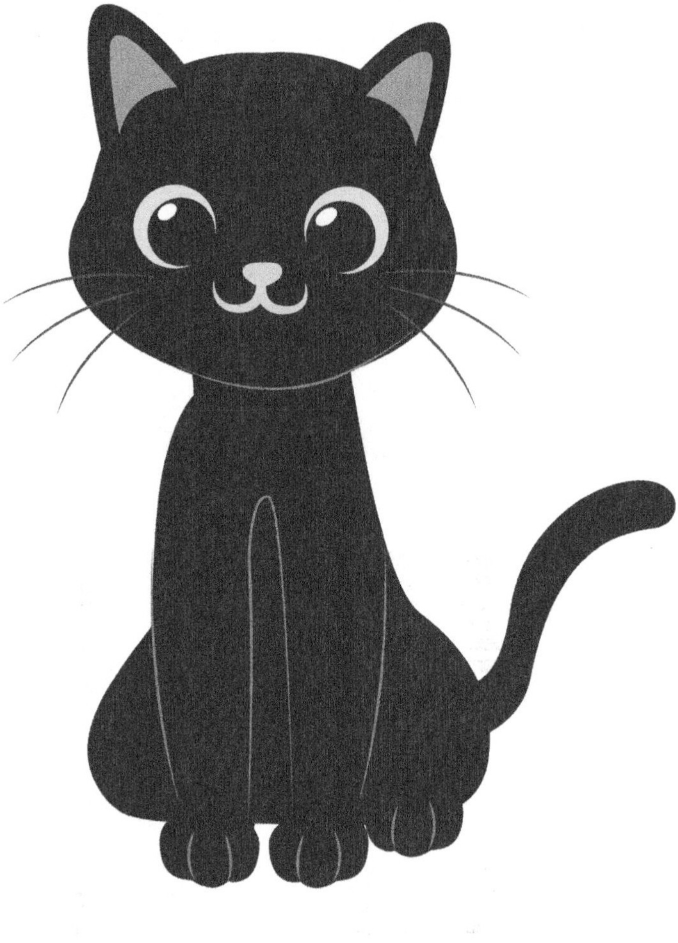

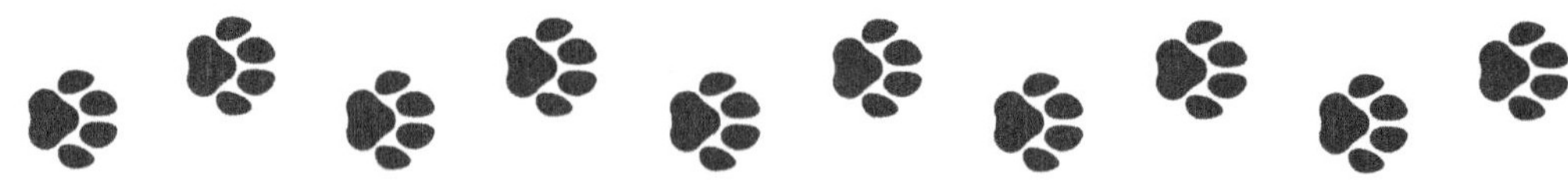

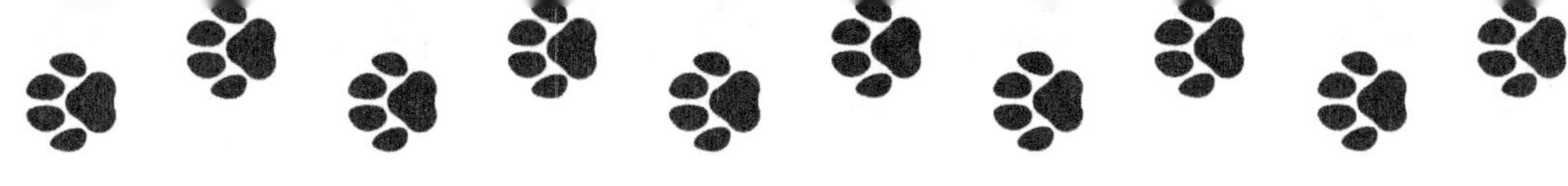

## GOALS

| Goal:

| Motivation

| Action Steps

#1

#2

#3

#4

#5

| Achieved:

| Reward:

| Goal:

| Motivation

| Action Steps

#1

#2

#3

#4

#5

| Achieved:

| Reward:

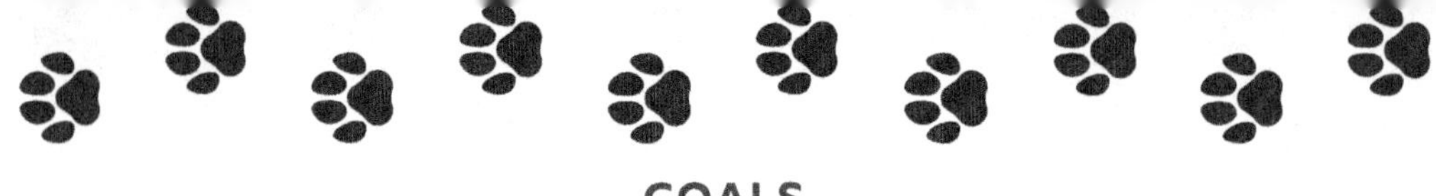

## GOALS

| Goal:

| Motivation

| Action Steps

#1

#2

#3

#4

#5

| Achieved:

| Reward:

| Goal:

| Motivation

| Action Steps

#1

#2

#3

#4

#5

| Achieved:

| Reward:

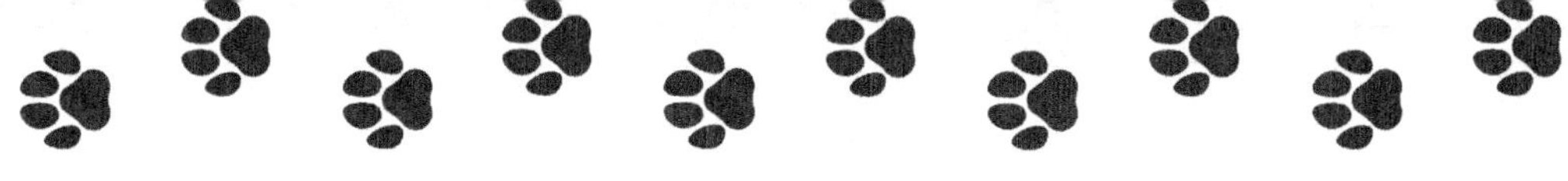

## GOALS

| Goal:

| Motivation

| Action Steps

#1

#2

#3

#4

#5

| Achieved:

| Reward:

| Goal:

| Motivation

| Action Steps

#1

#2

#3

#4

#5

| Achieved:

| Reward:

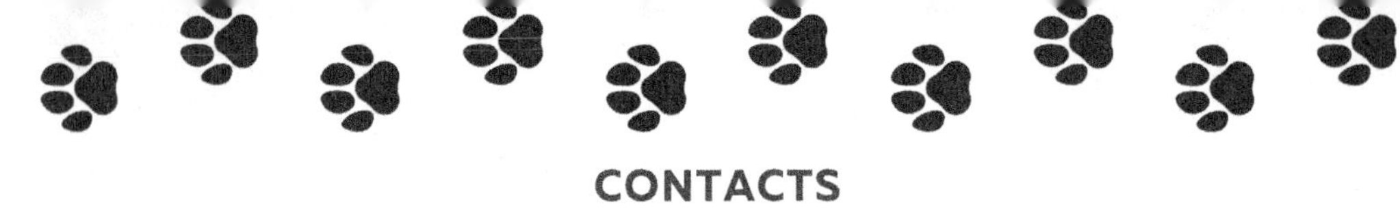

## CONTACTS

| Name | Phone | Email |
| --- | --- | --- |
| | | |

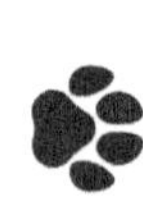
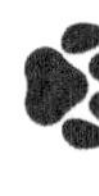

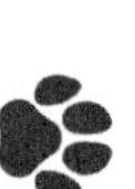
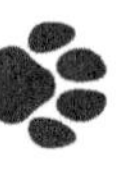
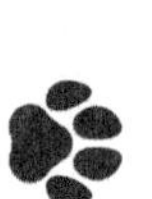
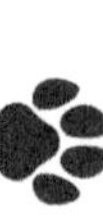

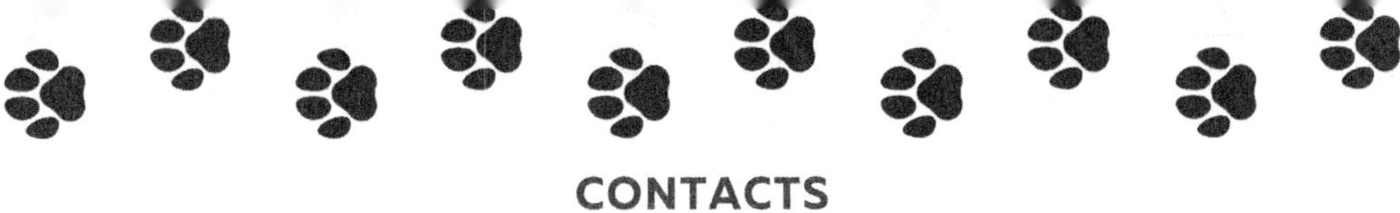

## CONTACTS

| Name | Phone | Email |
| --- | --- | --- |
| | | |

 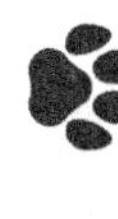 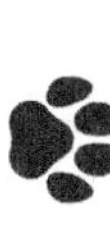 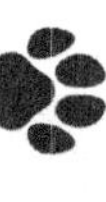 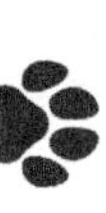   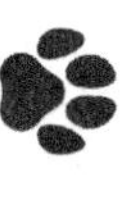  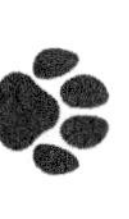

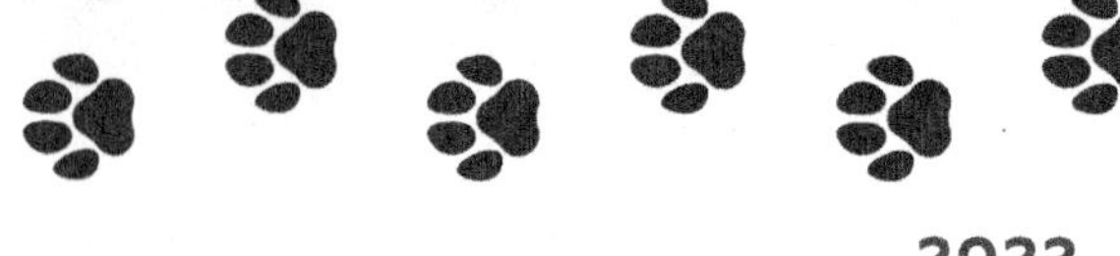

# 2022

## JANUARY

| M | T | W | T | F | S | S |
|---|---|---|---|---|---|---|
| | | | | | 1 | 2 |
| 3 | 4 | 5 | 6 | 7 | 8 | 9 |
| 10 | 11 | 12 | 13 | 14 | 15 | 16 |
| 17 | 18 | 19 | 20 | 21 | 22 | 23 |
| 24 | 25 | 26 | 27 | 28 | 29 | 30 |
| 31 | | | | | | |

## FEBRUARY

| M | T | W | T | F | S | S |
|---|---|---|---|---|---|---|
| | 1 | 2 | 3 | 4 | 5 | 6 |
| 7 | 8 | 9 | 10 | 11 | 12 | 13 |
| 14 | 15 | 16 | 17 | 18 | 19 | 20 |
| 21 | 22 | 23 | 24 | 25 | 26 | 27 |
| 28 | | | | | | |

## MARCH

| M | T | W | T | F | S | S |
|---|---|---|---|---|---|---|
| | 1 | 2 | 3 | 4 | 5 | 6 |
| 7 | 8 | 9 | 10 | 11 | 12 | 13 |
| 14 | 15 | 16 | 17 | 18 | 19 | 20 |
| 21 | 22 | 23 | 24 | 25 | 26 | 27 |
| 28 | 29 | 30 | 31 | | | |

## APRIL

| M | T | W | T | F | S | S |
|---|---|---|---|---|---|---|
| | | | | 1 | 2 | 3 |
| 4 | 5 | 6 | 7 | 8 | 9 | 10 |
| 11 | 12 | 13 | 14 | 15 | 16 | 17 |
| 18 | 19 | 20 | 21 | 22 | 23 | 24 |
| 25 | 26 | 27 | 28 | 29 | 30 | |

## MAY

| M | T | W | T | F | S | S |
|---|---|---|---|---|---|---|
| | | | | | | 1 |
| 2 | 3 | 4 | 5 | 6 | 7 | 8 |
| 9 | 10 | 11 | 12 | 13 | 14 | 15 |
| 16 | 17 | 18 | 19 | 20 | 21 | 22 |
| 23 | 24 | 25 | 26 | 27 | 28 | 29 |
| 30 | 31 | | | | | |

## JUNE

| M | T | W | T | F | S | S |
|---|---|---|---|---|---|---|
| | | 1 | 2 | 3 | 4 | 5 |
| 6 | 7 | 8 | 9 | 10 | 11 | 12 |
| 13 | 14 | 15 | 16 | 17 | 18 | 19 |
| 20 | 21 | 22 | 23 | 24 | 25 | 26 |
| 27 | 28 | 29 | 30 | | | |

## JULY

| M | T | W | T | F | S | S |
|---|---|---|---|---|---|---|
| | | | | 1 | 2 | 3 |
| 4 | 5 | 6 | 7 | 8 | 9 | 10 |
| 11 | 12 | 13 | 14 | 15 | 16 | 17 |
| 18 | 19 | 20 | 21 | 22 | 23 | 24 |
| 25 | 26 | 27 | 28 | 29 | 30 | 31 |

## AUGUST

| M | T | W | T | F | S | S |
|---|---|---|---|---|---|---|
| 1 | 2 | 3 | 4 | 5 | 6 | 7 |
| 8 | 9 | 10 | 11 | 12 | 13 | 14 |
| 15 | 16 | 17 | 18 | 19 | 20 | 21 |
| 22 | 23 | 24 | 25 | 26 | 27 | 28 |
| 29 | 30 | 31 | | | | |

## SEPTEMBER

| M | T | W | T | F | S | S |
|---|---|---|---|---|---|---|
| | | | 1 | 2 | 3 | 4 |
| 5 | 6 | 7 | 8 | 9 | 10 | 11 |
| 12 | 13 | 14 | 15 | 16 | 17 | 18 |
| 19 | 20 | 21 | 22 | 23 | 24 | 25 |
| 26 | 27 | 28 | 29 | 30 | | |

## OCTOBER

| M | T | W | T | F | S | S |
|---|---|---|---|---|---|---|
| | | | | | 1 | 2 |
| 3 | 4 | 5 | 6 | 7 | 8 | 9 |
| 10 | 11 | 12 | 13 | 14 | 15 | 16 |
| 17 | 18 | 19 | 20 | 21 | 22 | 23 |
| 24 | 25 | 26 | 27 | 28 | 29 | 30 |
| 31 | | | | | | |

## NOVEMBER

| M | T | W | T | F | S | S |
|---|---|---|---|---|---|---|
| | 1 | 2 | 3 | 4 | 5 | 6 |
| 7 | 8 | 9 | 10 | 11 | 12 | 13 |
| 14 | 15 | 16 | 17 | 18 | 19 | 20 |
| 21 | 22 | 23 | 24 | 25 | 26 | 27 |
| 28 | 29 | 30 | | | | |

## DECEMBER

| M | T | W | T | F | S | S |
|---|---|---|---|---|---|---|
| | | | 1 | 2 | 3 | 4 |
| 5 | 6 | 7 | 8 | 9 | 10 | 11 |
| 12 | 13 | 14 | 15 | 16 | 17 | 18 |
| 19 | 20 | 21 | 22 | 23 | 24 | 25 |
| 26 | 27 | 28 | 29 | 30 | 31 | |

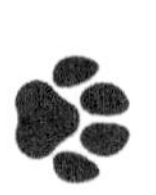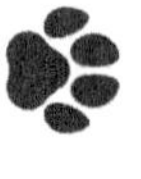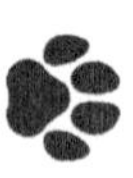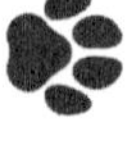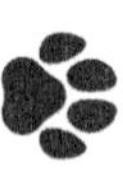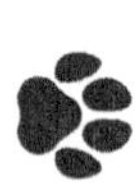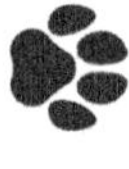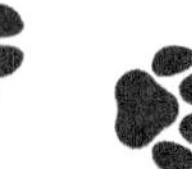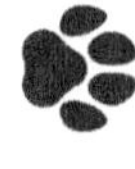

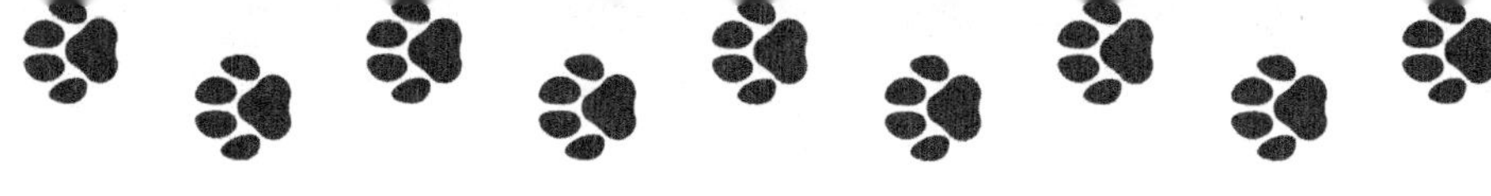

## HOLIDAYS

| Date | Holiday |
|---|---|
| 1 January 2022 | New Year's Day |
| 3 January 2022 | New Year's Day observed |
| 1 March 2022 | St. David's Day |
| 15 April 2022 | Good Friday |
| 17 April 2022 | Easter Sunday |
| 18 April 2022 | Easter Monday |
| 25 April 2022 | St. George's Day |
| 2 May 2022 | Early May Bank Holiday |
| 2 June 2022 | Spring Bank Holiday |
| 3 June 2022 | Queen's Platinum Jubilee |
| 11 June 2022 | Queen's Birthday |
| 29 August 2022 | Summer Bank Holiday |
| 31 October 2022 | Halloween |
| 5 November 2022 | Guy Fawkes Day |
| 13 November 2022 | Remembrance Sunday |
| 25 December 2022 | Christmas Day |
| 26 December 2022 | Boxing Day |
| 27 December 2022 | Substitute Bank Holiday for Christmas Day |
| 31 December 2022 | New Year's Eve |

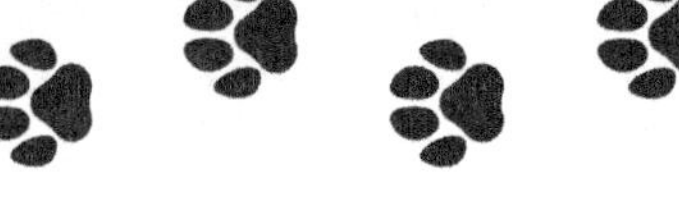

## JANUARY

| Monday | Tuesday | Wednesday | Thursday |
| --- | --- | --- | --- |
| | | | |
| 3 New Year's Day observed | 4 | 5 | 6 |
| 10 | 11 | 12 | 13 |
| 17 | 18 | 19 | 20 |
| 24 | 25 | 26 | 27 |
| 31 | | | |

| Friday | Saturday | Sunday |
|---|---|---|
| | 1 New Year's Day | 2 |
| 7 | 8 | 9 |
| 14 | 15 | 16 |
| 21 | 22 | 23 |
| 28 | 29 | 30 |

Goals

To Do

Reminder

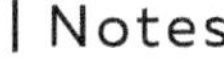

Notes

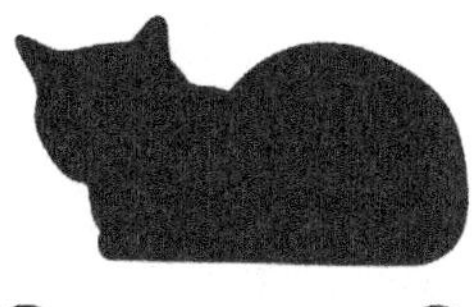

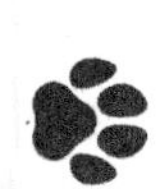
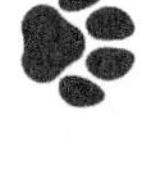
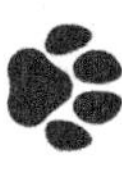
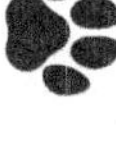
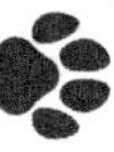
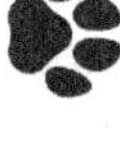
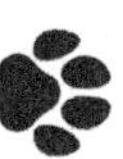

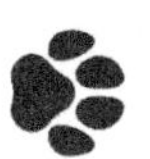
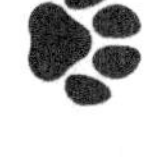

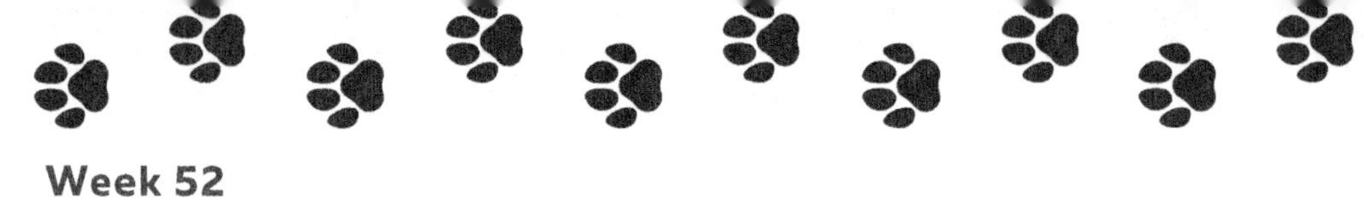

# Week 52

## 27 | Monday

## 28 | Tuesday

## 29 | Wednesday

## 30 | Thursday

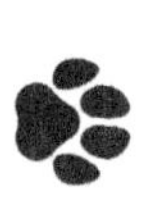 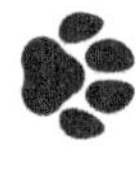 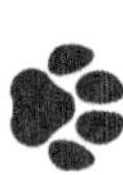 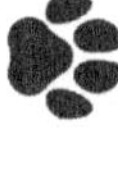 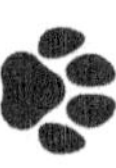 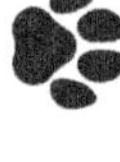 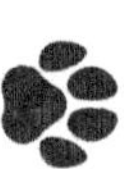 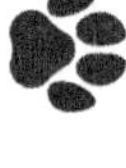 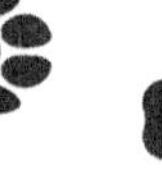 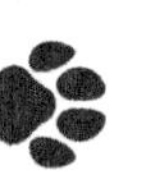 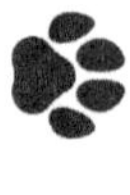

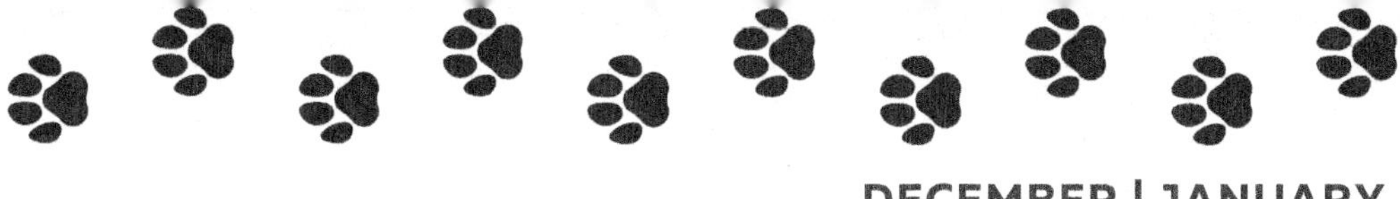



31 | Friday — New Year's Eve

1 | Saturday — New Year's Day

2 | Sunday

Notes

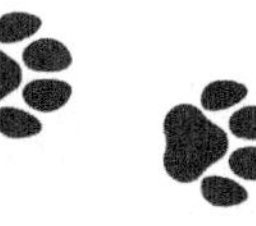
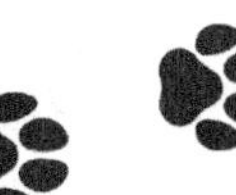
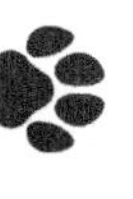
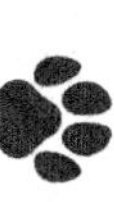
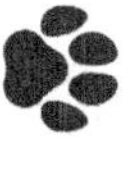
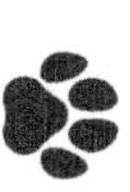
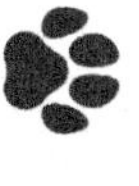
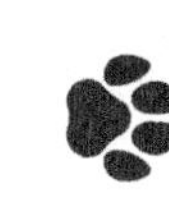
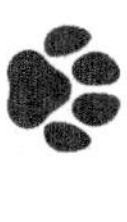

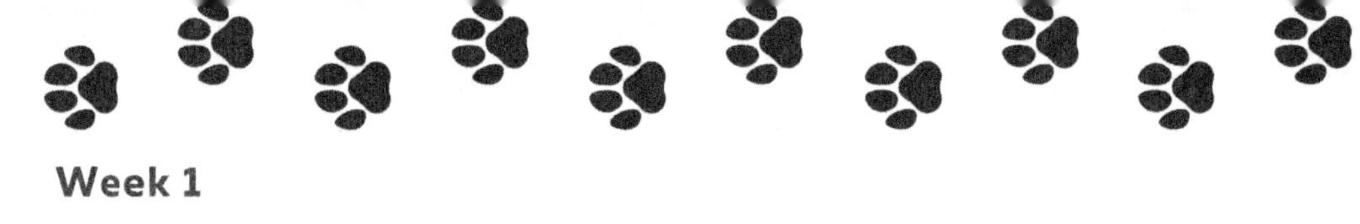

## Week 1

3 | Monday New Year's Day observed

4 | Tuesday

5 | Wednesday

6 | Thursday

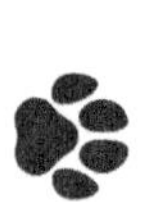
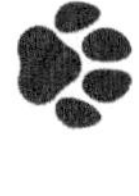

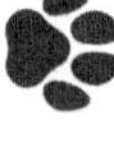
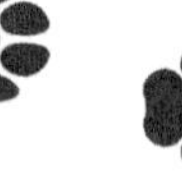
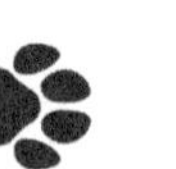
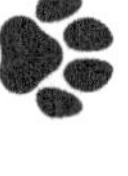
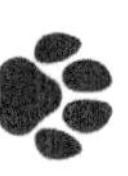
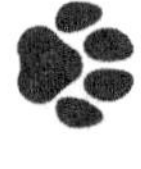
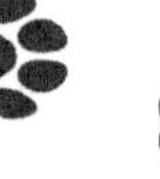
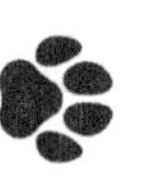
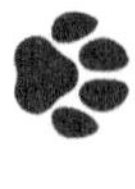

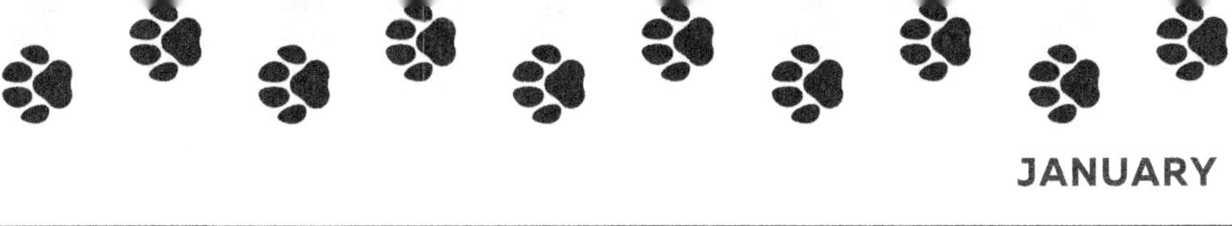



7 | Friday

8 | Saturday

9 | Sunday

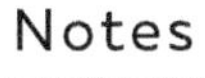

Notes

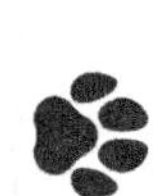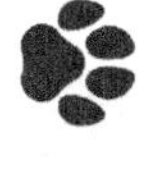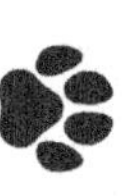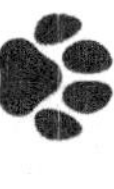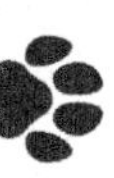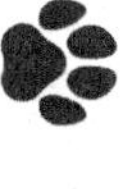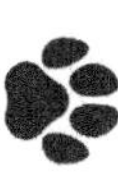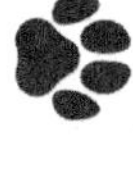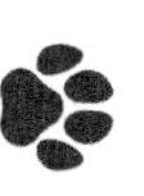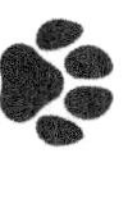

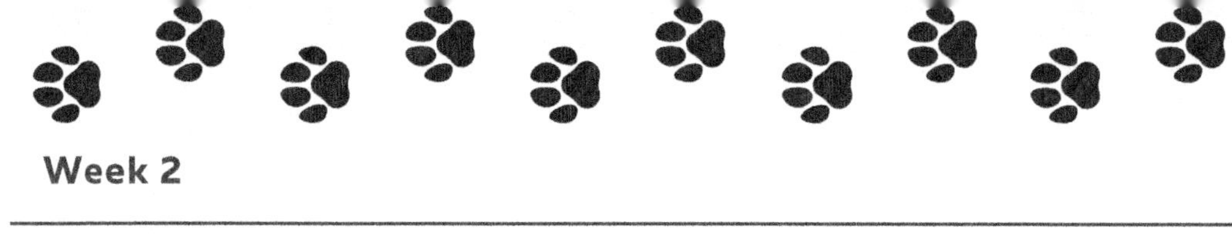

## Week 2

### 10 | Monday

### 11 | Tuesday

### 12 | Wednesday

### 13 | Thursday

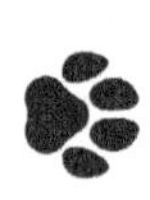
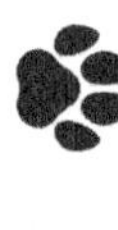
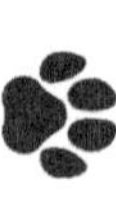
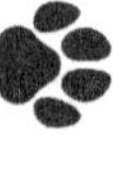

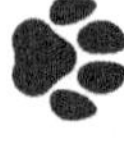
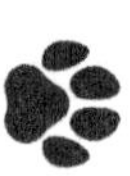
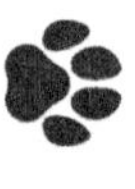
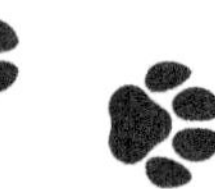
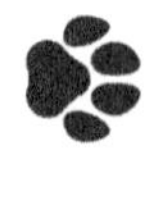

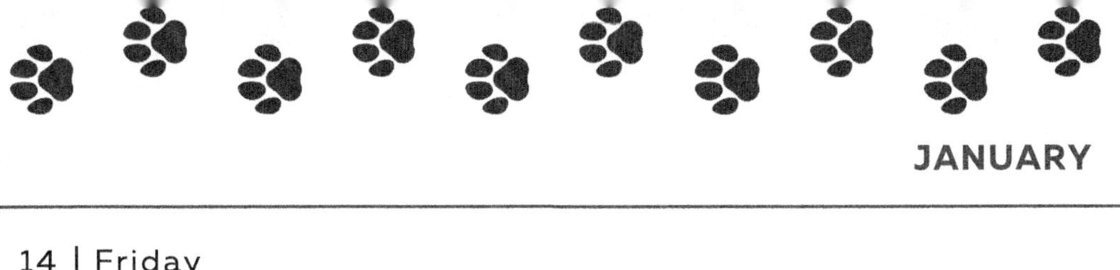



## 14 | Friday

## 15 | Saturday

## 16 | Sunday

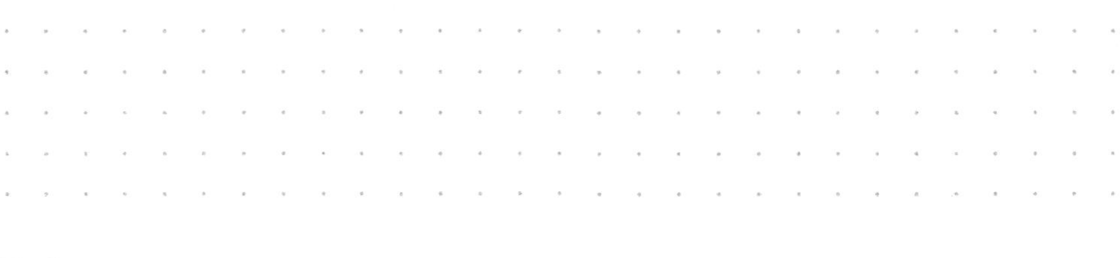

## Notes

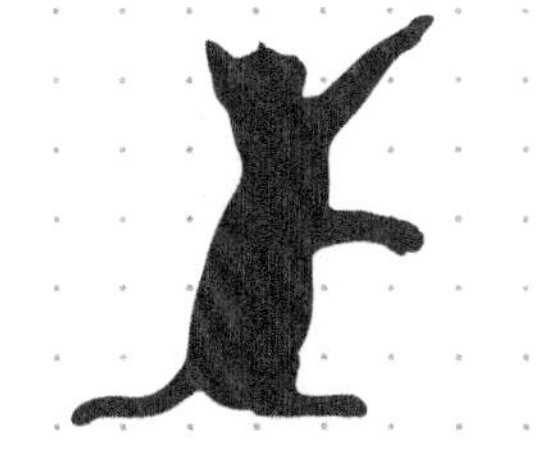

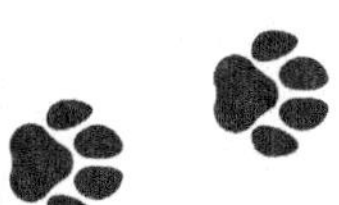
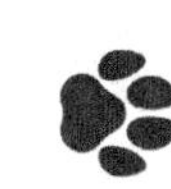
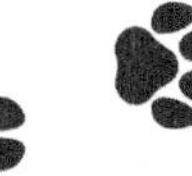
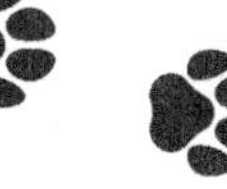
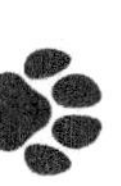
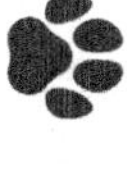
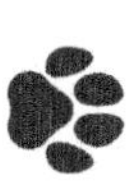
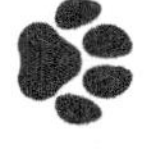
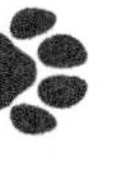
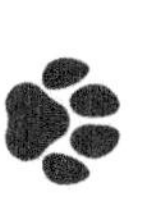
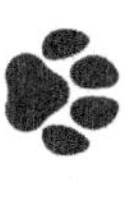

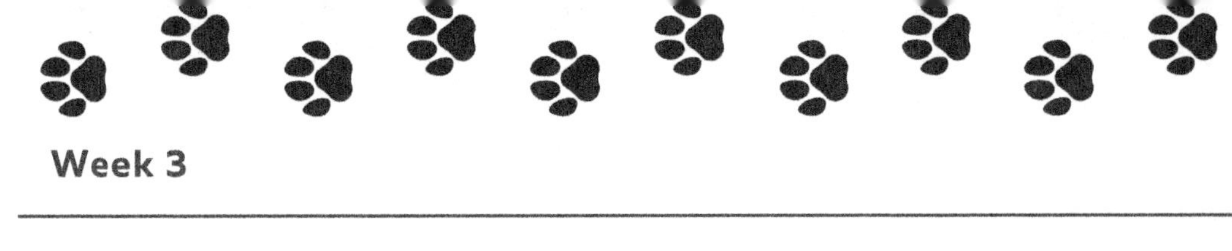

## Week 3

### 17 | Monday

### 18 | Tuesday

### 19 | Wednesday

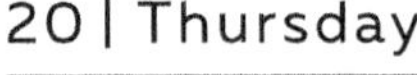

### 20 | Thursday

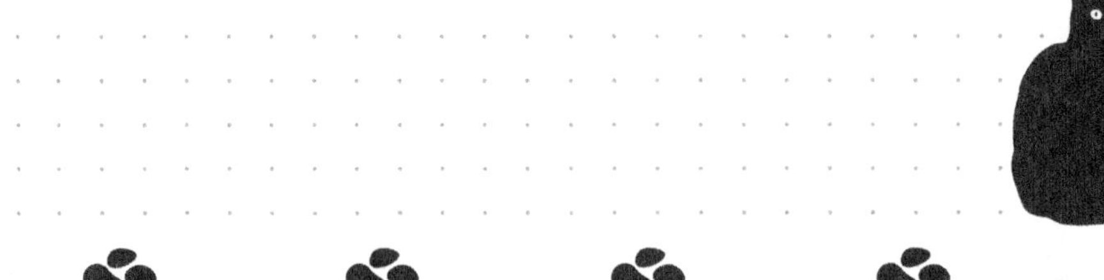

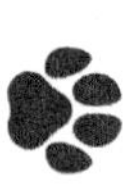 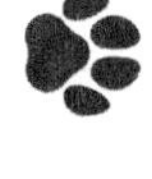 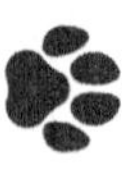 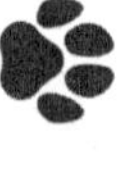 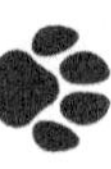 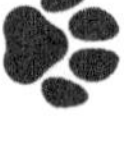 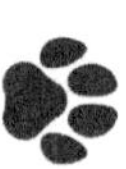 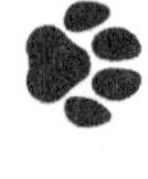 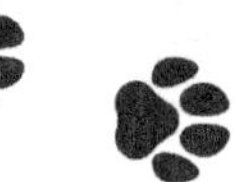 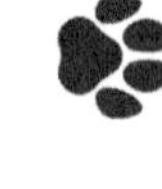

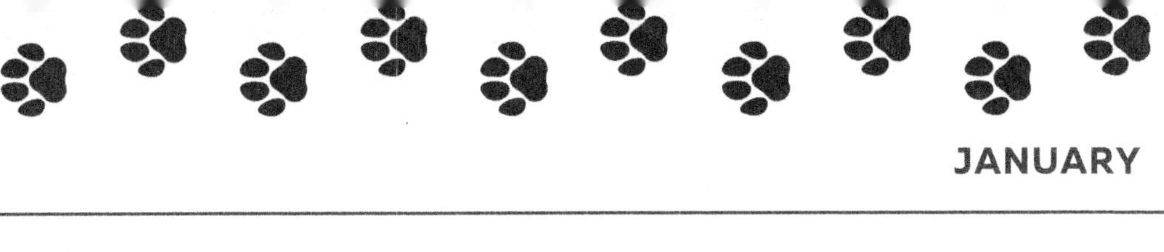



21 | Friday

22 | Saturday

23 | Sunday

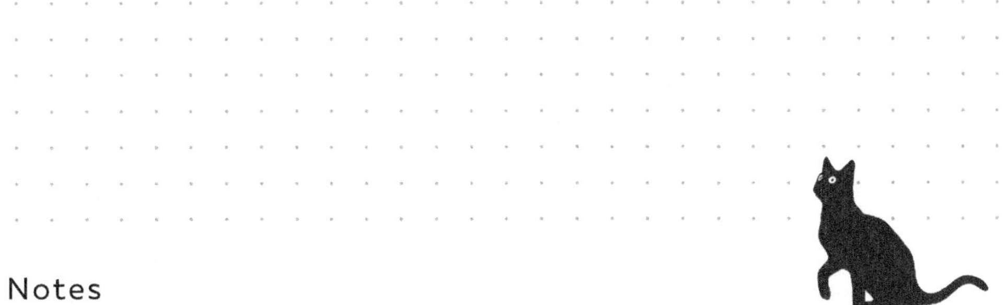

Notes

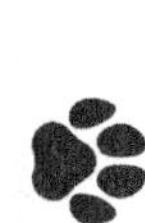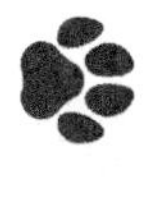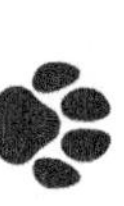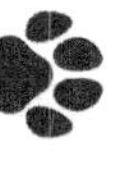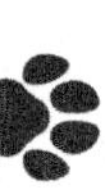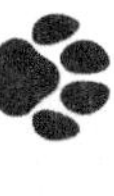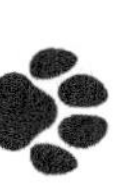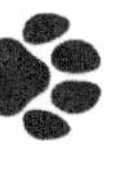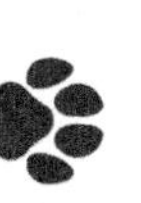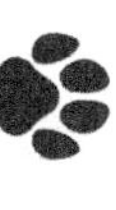

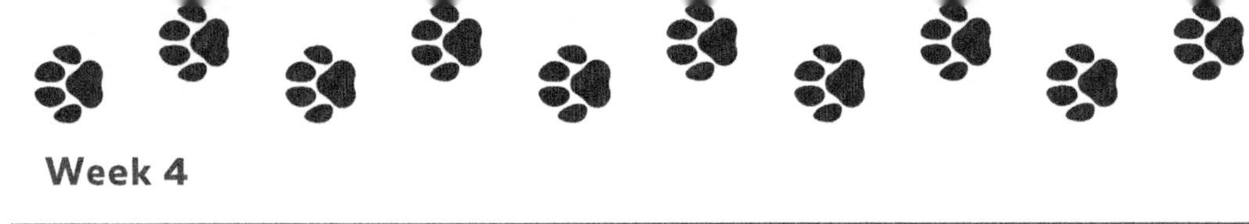

## Week 4

### 24 | Monday

### 25 | Tuesday

### 26 | Wednesday

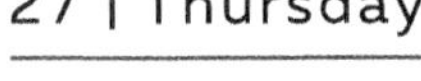

### 27 | Thursday

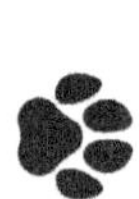
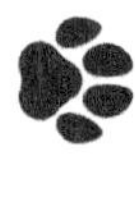
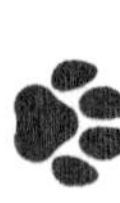
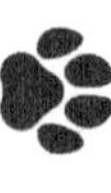
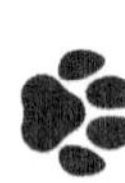
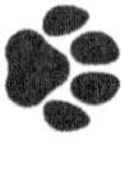
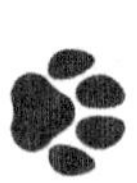
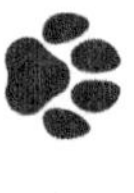
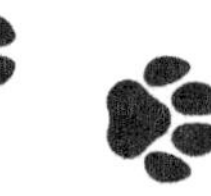
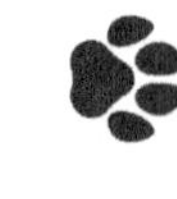

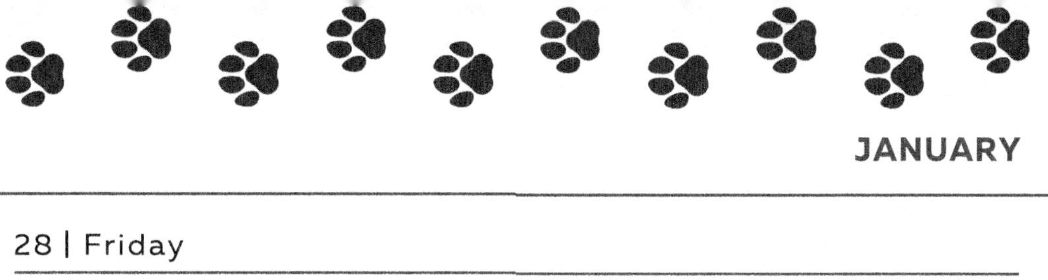



28 | Friday

29 | Saturday

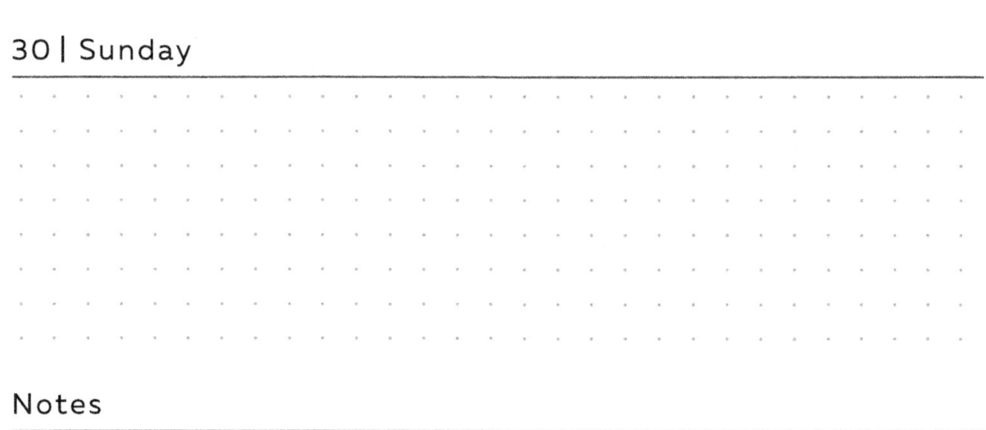

30 | Sunday

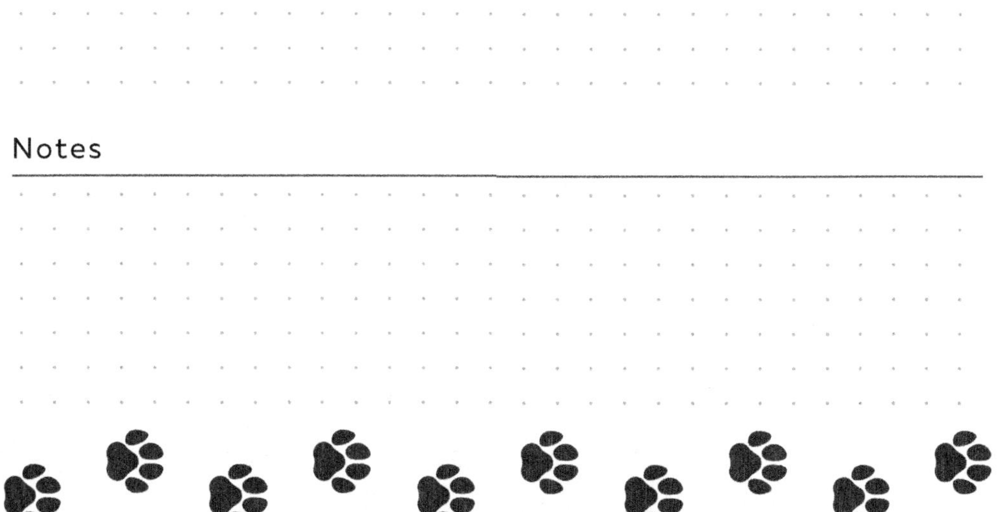

Notes

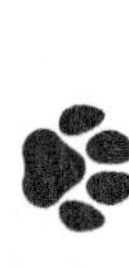
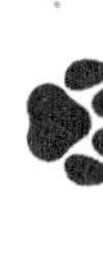
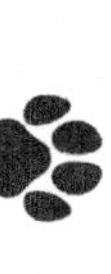
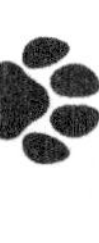
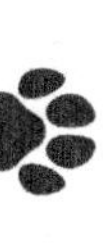
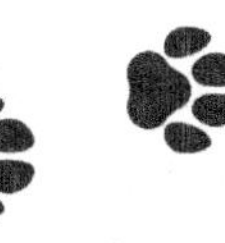

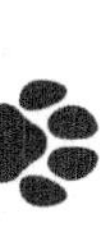
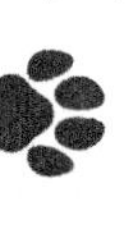

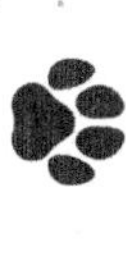

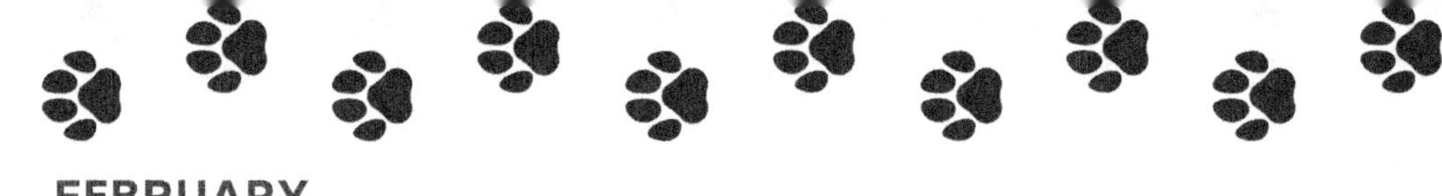

# FEBRUARY

| Monday | Tuesday | Wednesday | Thursday |
|---|---|---|---|
| | 1 | 2 | 3 |
| 7 | 8 | 9 | 10 |
| 14 Valentine's Day | 15 | 16 | 17 |
| 21 | 22 | 23 | 24 |
| 28 | | | |

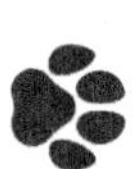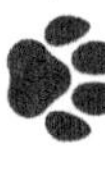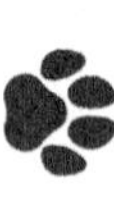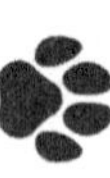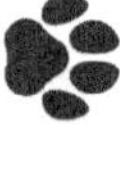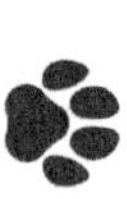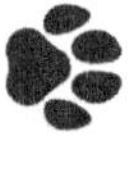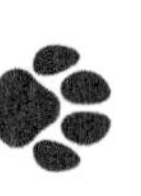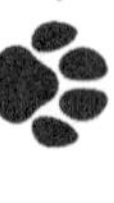

| Friday | Saturday | Sunday |
| --- | --- | --- |
| 4 | 5 | 6 |
| 11 | 12 | 13 |
| 18 | 19 | 20 |
| 25 | 26 | 27 |

Goals

To Do

Reminder

Notes

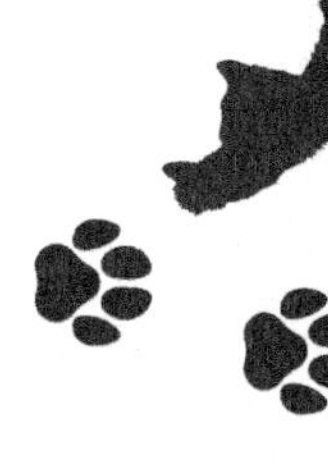

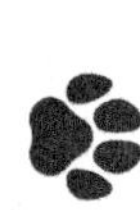
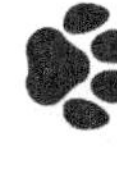
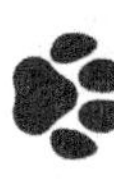
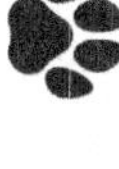
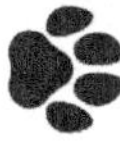
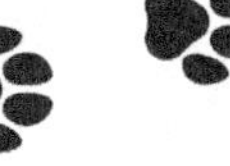
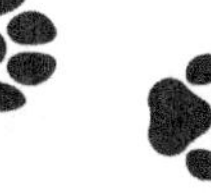
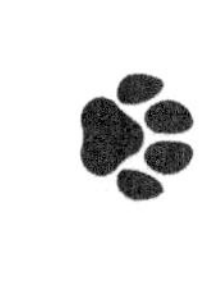

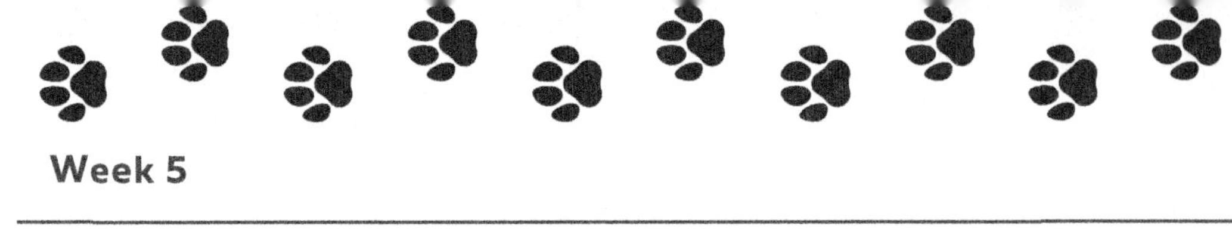

## Week 5

31 | Monday

1 | Tuesday

2 | Wednesday

3 | Thursday

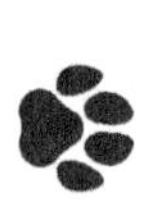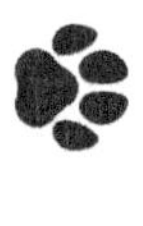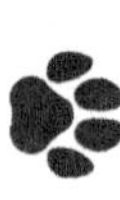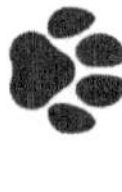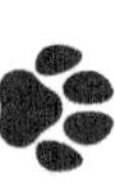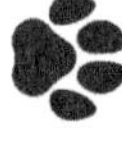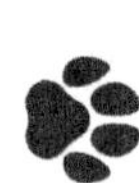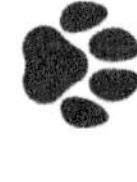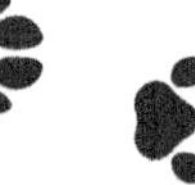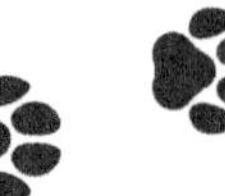

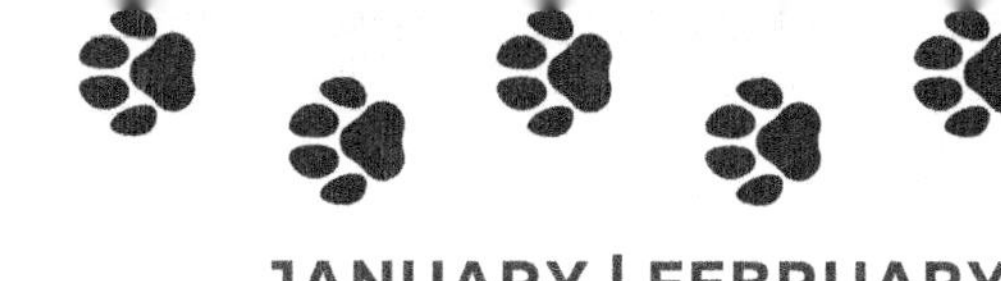



4 | Friday

5 | Saturday

6 | Sunday

Notes

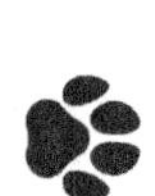
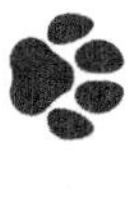
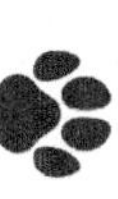
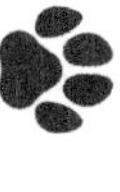
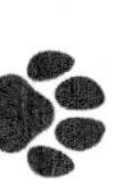
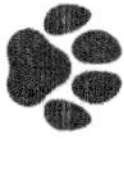
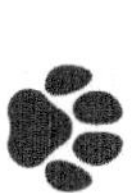
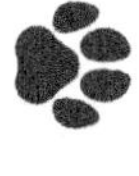
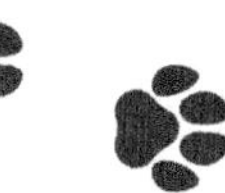
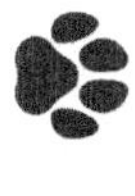

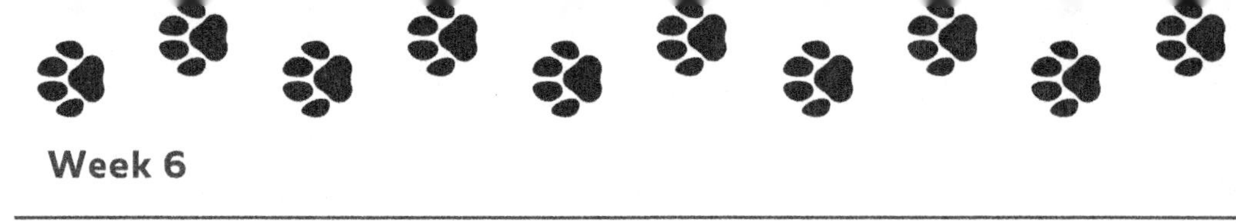

## Week 6

7 | Monday

8 | Tuesday

9 | Wednesday

10 | Thursday

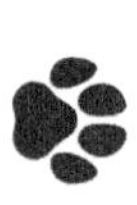
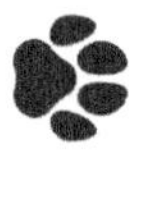
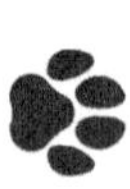
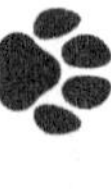
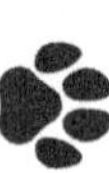
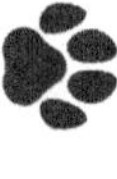
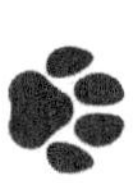
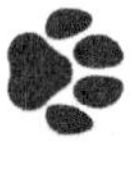
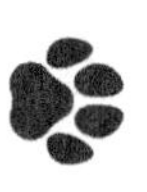
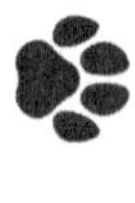

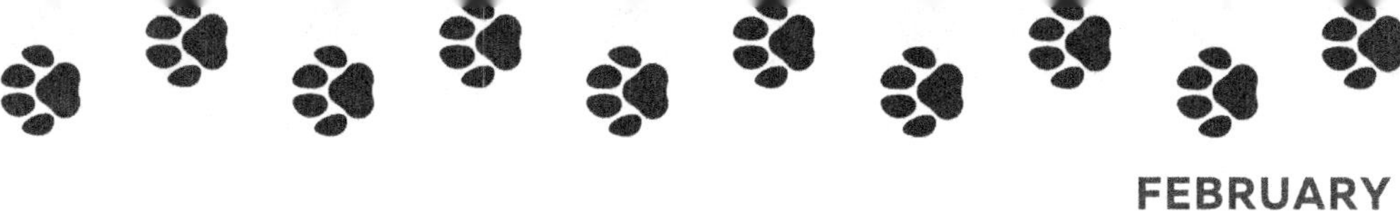



11 | Friday

12 | Saturday

13 | Sunday

Notes

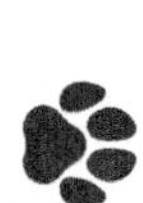
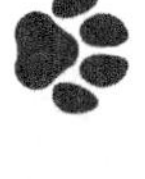
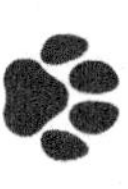

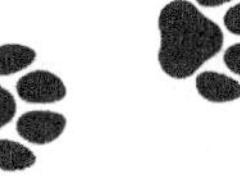
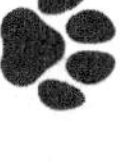
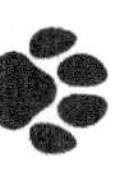
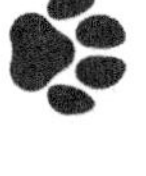
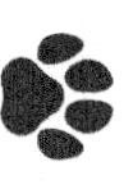
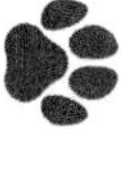

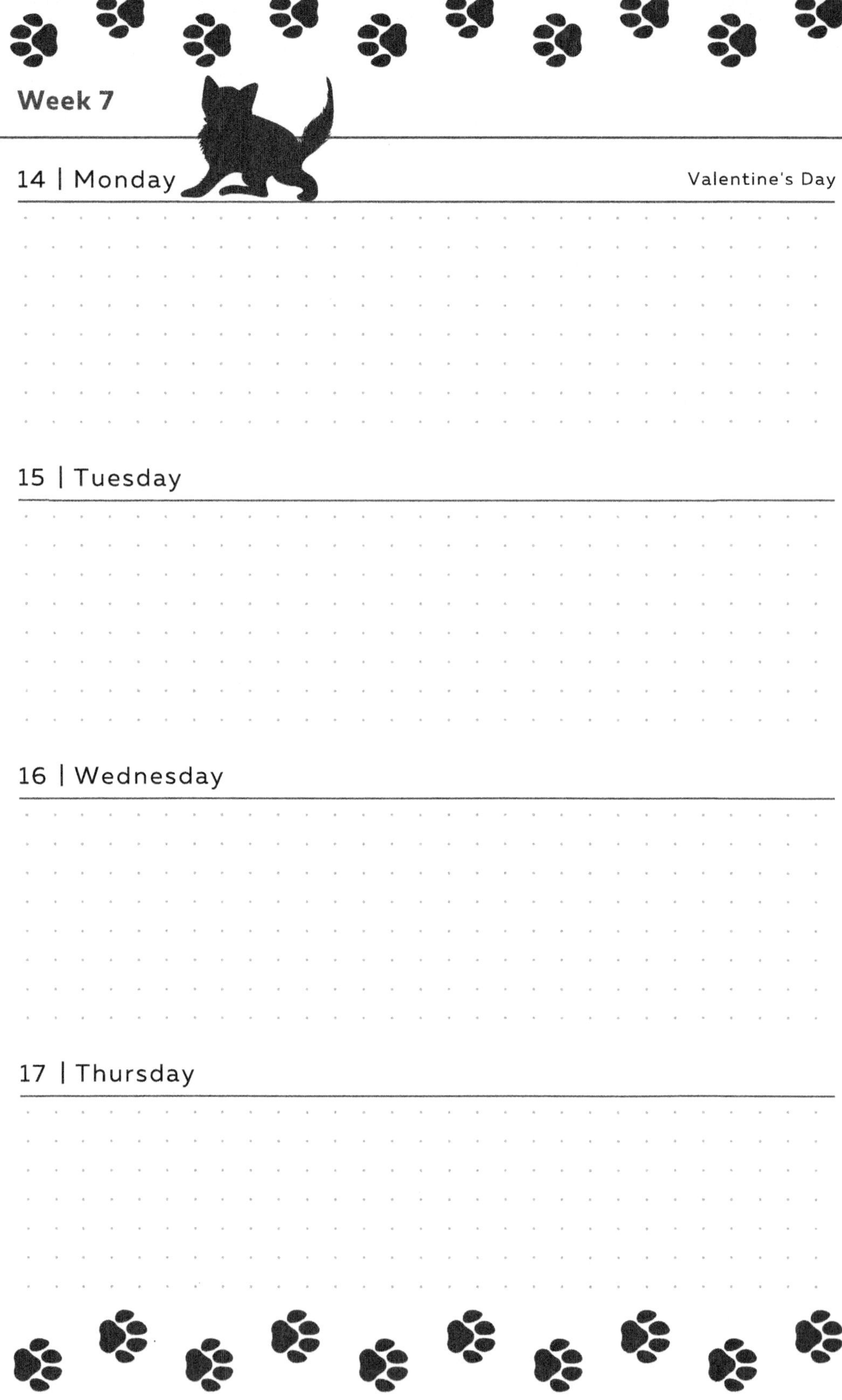

## Week 7

### 14 | Monday

Valentine's Day

### 15 | Tuesday

### 16 | Wednesday

### 17 | Thursday

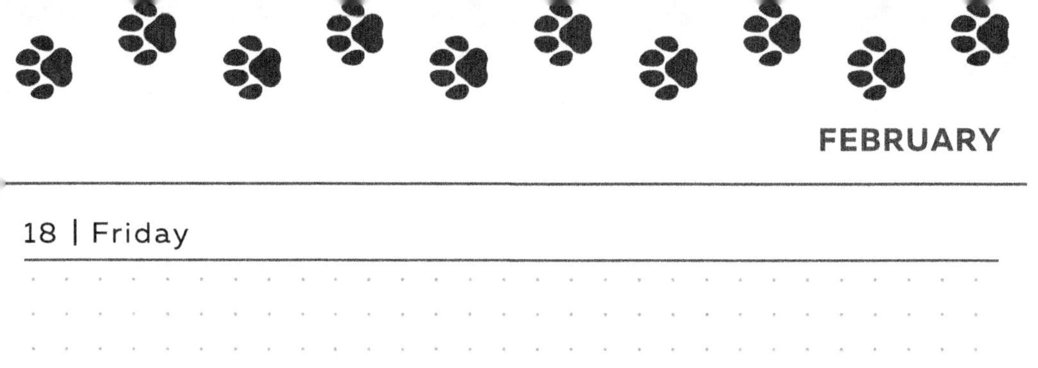

FEBRUARY

18 | Friday

19 | Saturday

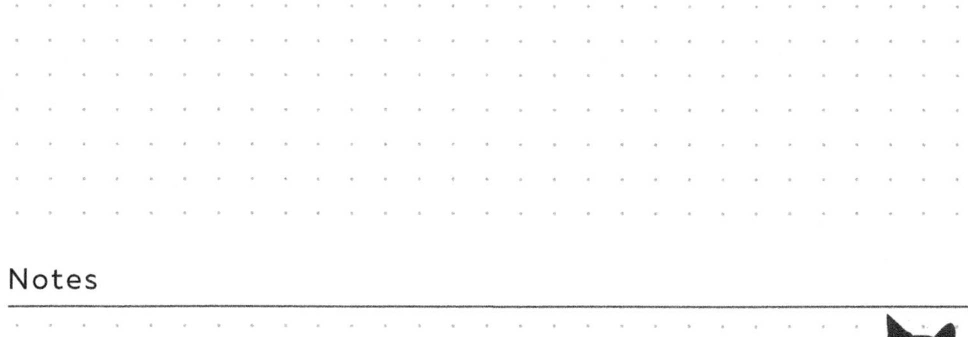

20 | Sunday

Notes

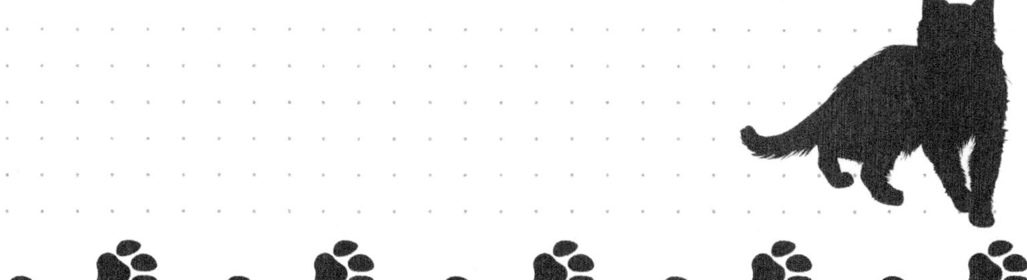

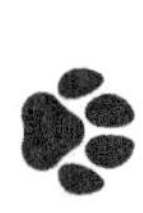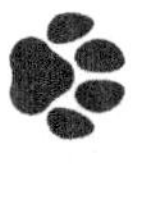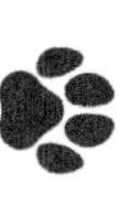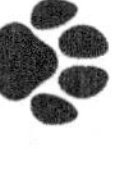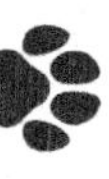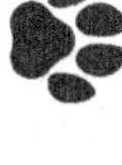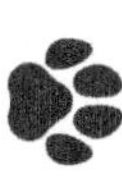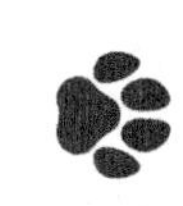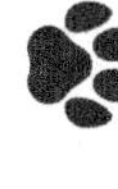

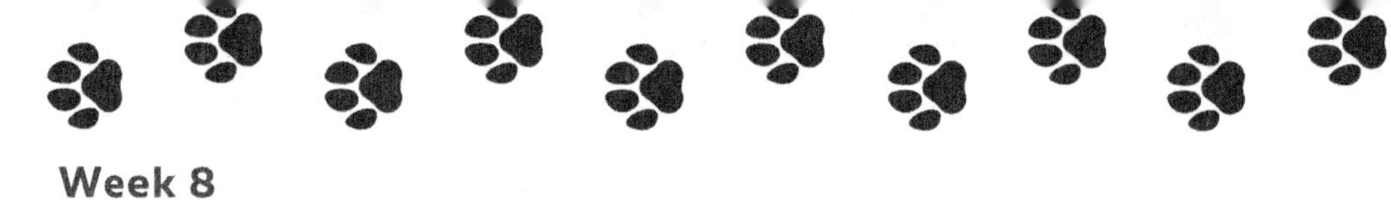

## Week 8

### 21 | Monday

### 22 | Tuesday

### 23 | Wednesday

### 24 | Thursday

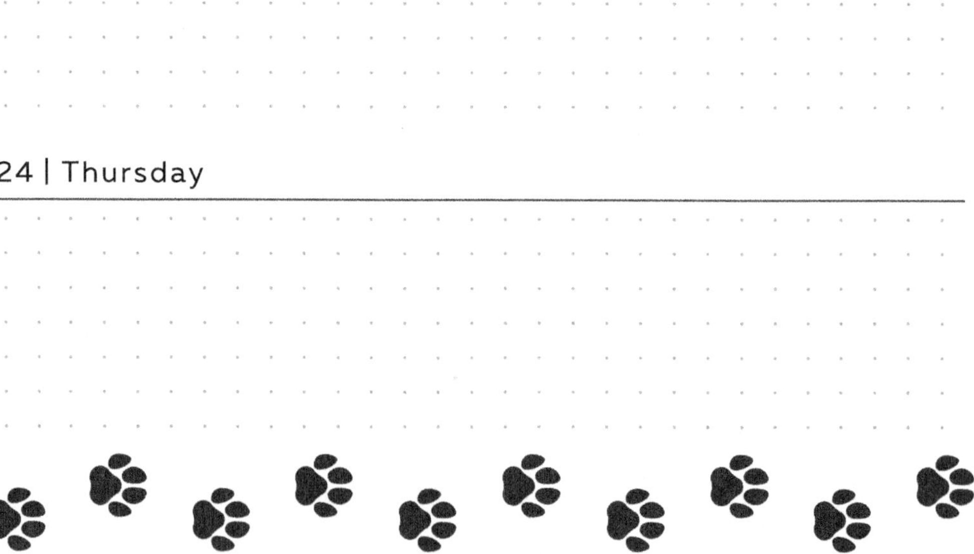

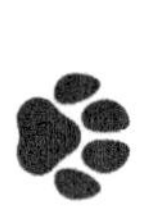
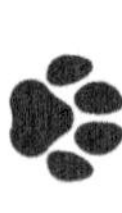
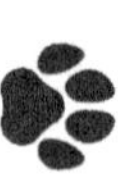
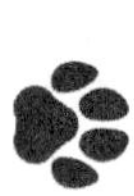
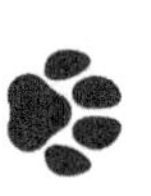
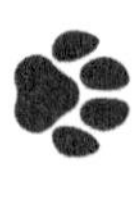

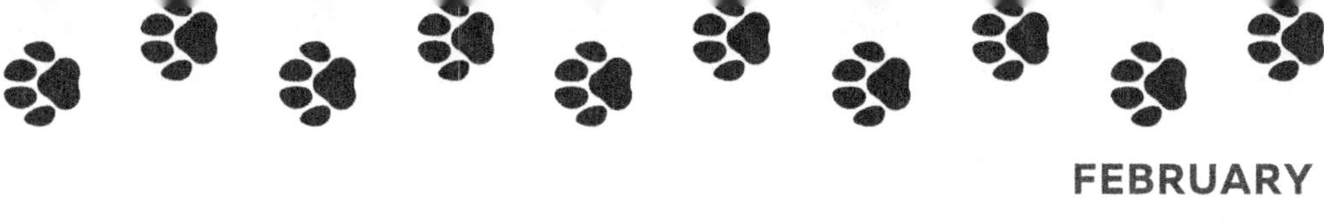



25 | Friday

26 | Saturday

27 | Sunday

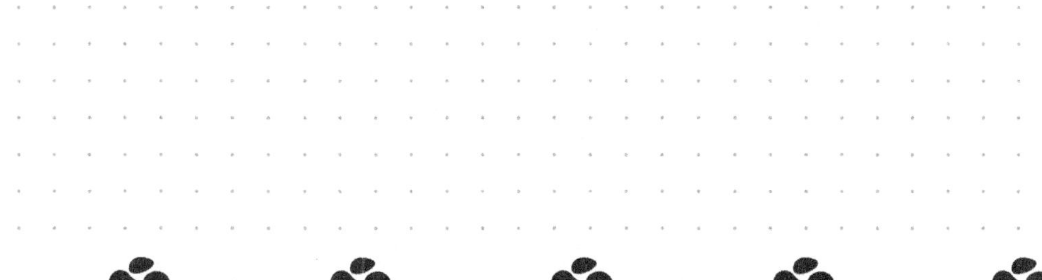

Notes

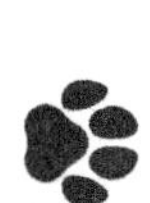
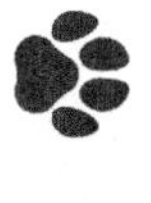
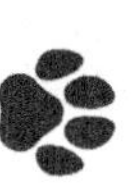
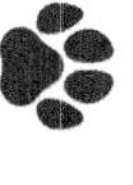
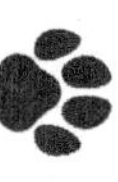
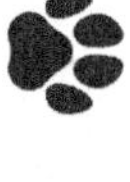
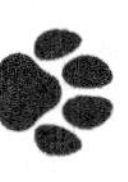
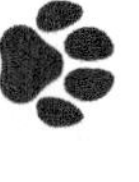
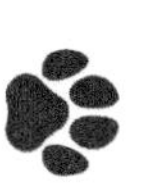
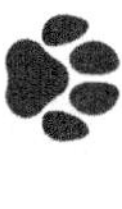

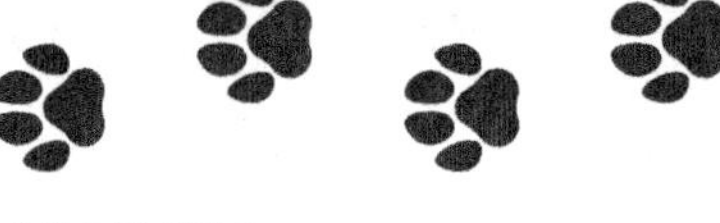

## MARCH

| Monday | Tuesday | Wednesday | Thursday |
| --- | --- | --- | --- |
| | 1 St. David's Day | 2 | 3 |
| 7 | 8 | 9 | 10 |
| 14 | 15 | 16 | 17 |
| 21 | 22 | 23 | 24 |
| 28 | 29 | 30 | 31 |

2022

| Friday | Saturday | Sunday |
| --- | --- | --- |
| 4 | 5 | 6 |
| 11 | 12 | 13 |
| 18 | 19 | 20 |
| 25 | 26 | 27 |

Goals

To Do

Reminder

Notes

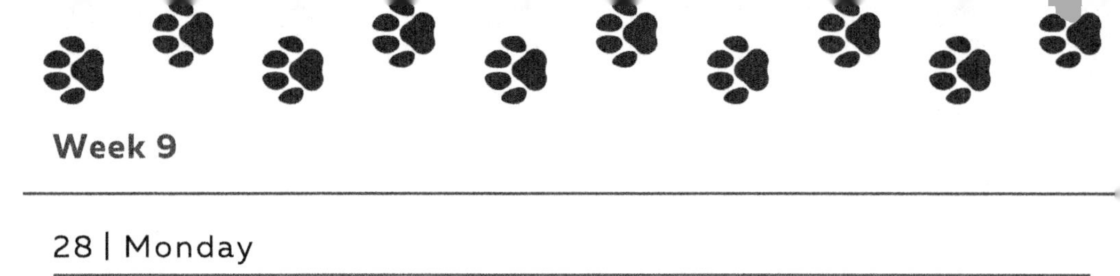

## Week 9

### 28 | Monday

### 1 | Tuesday

St. David's Day

### 2 | Wednesday

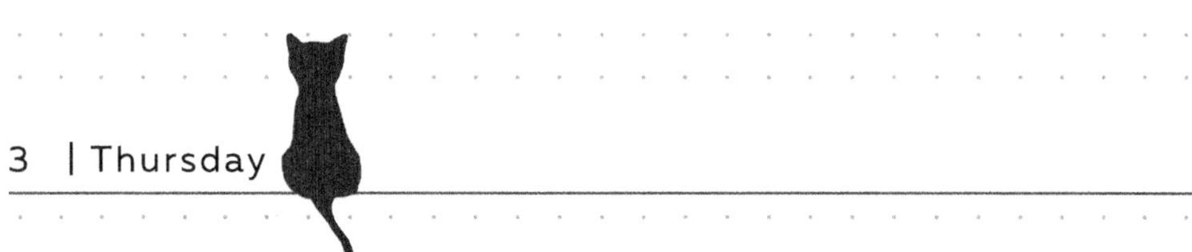

### 3 | Thursday

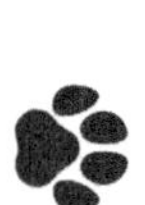
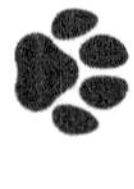
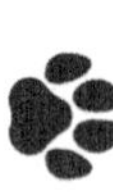

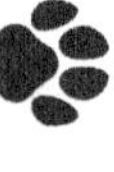
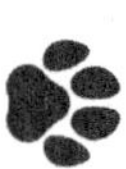
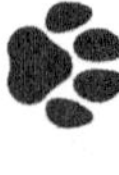
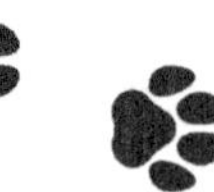
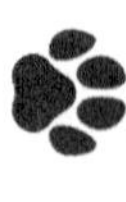

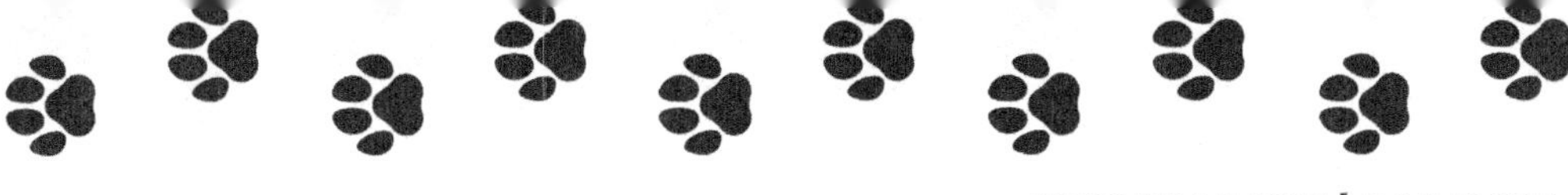



4 | Friday

5 | Saturday

6 | Sunday

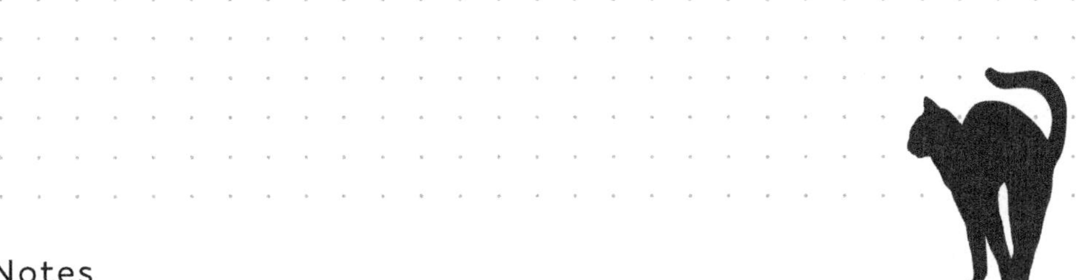

Notes

 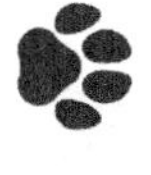 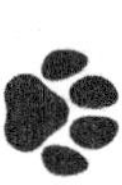 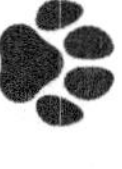 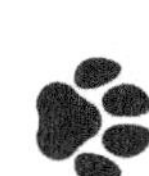 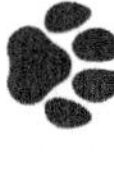 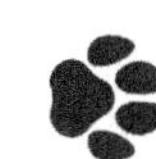 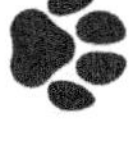 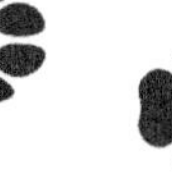 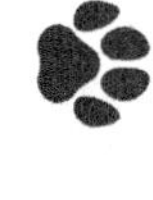

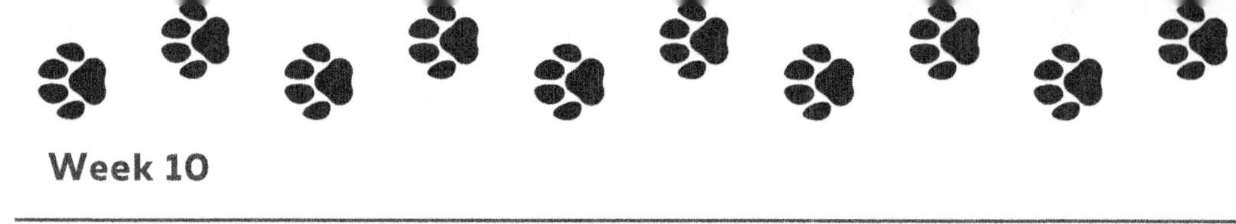

## Week 10

7 | Monday

8 | Tuesday

9 | Wednesday

10 | Thursday

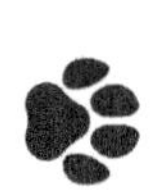
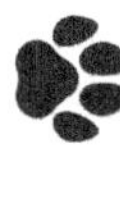
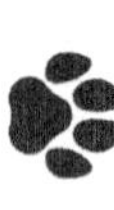

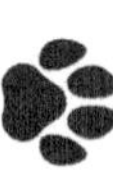
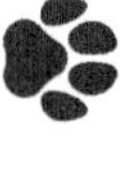
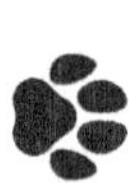
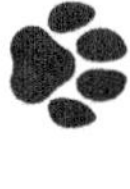
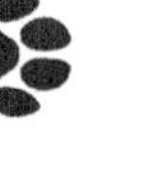
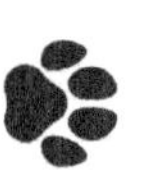
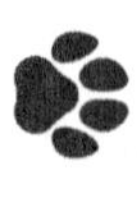

11 | Friday

12 | Saturday

13 | Sunday

Notes

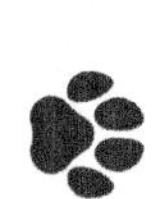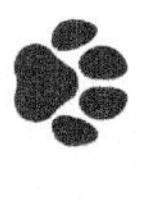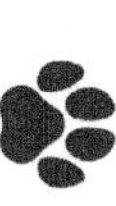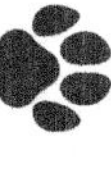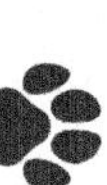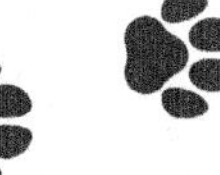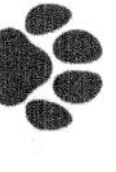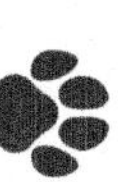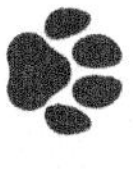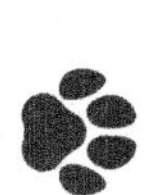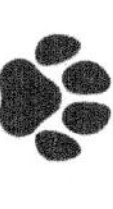

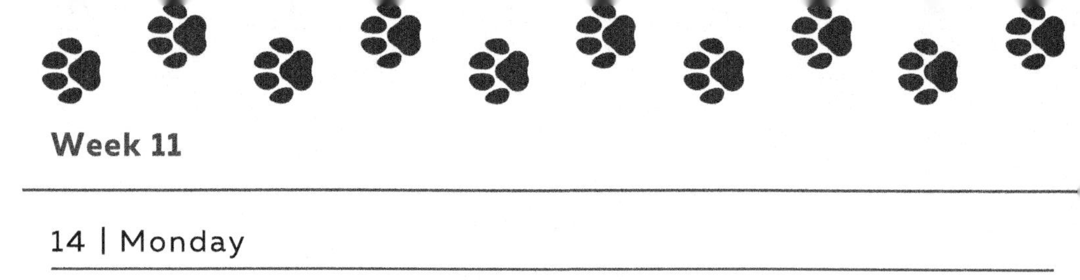

## Week 11

### 14 | Monday

### 15 | Tuesday

### 16 | Wednesday

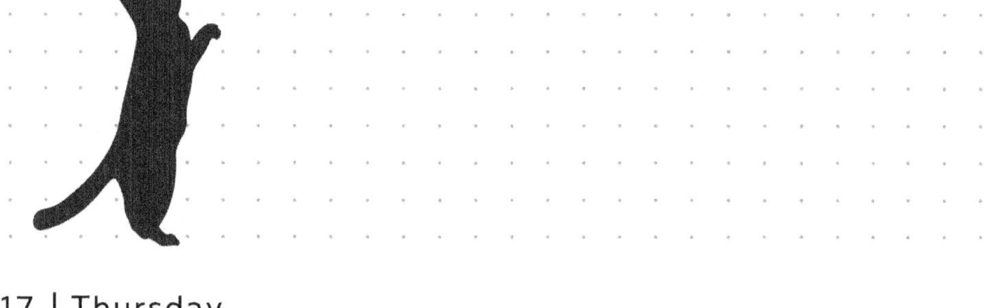

### 17 | Thursday

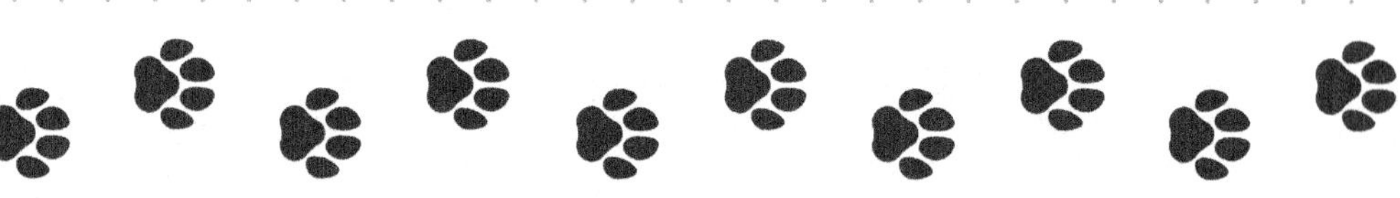

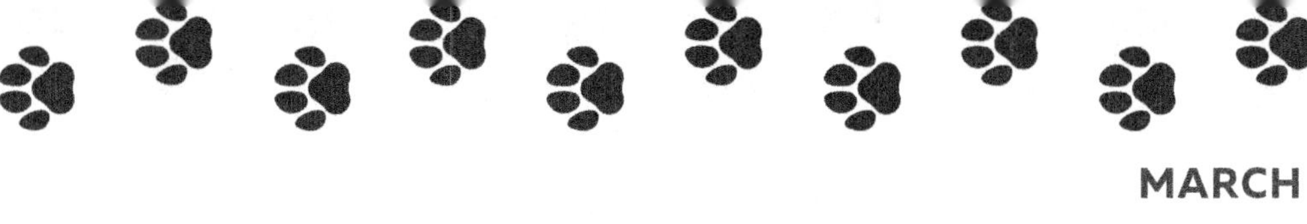



18 | Friday

19 | Saturday

20 | Sunday

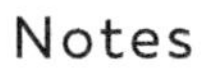

Notes

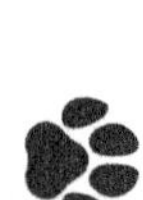
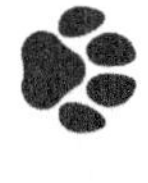
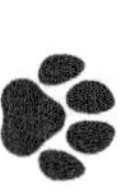
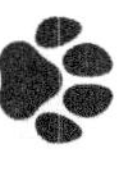
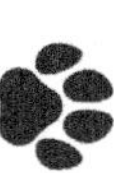
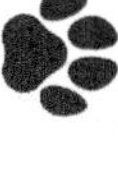
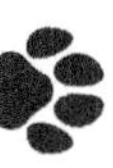
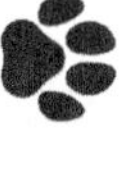
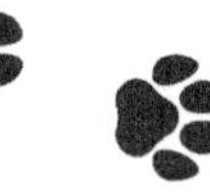

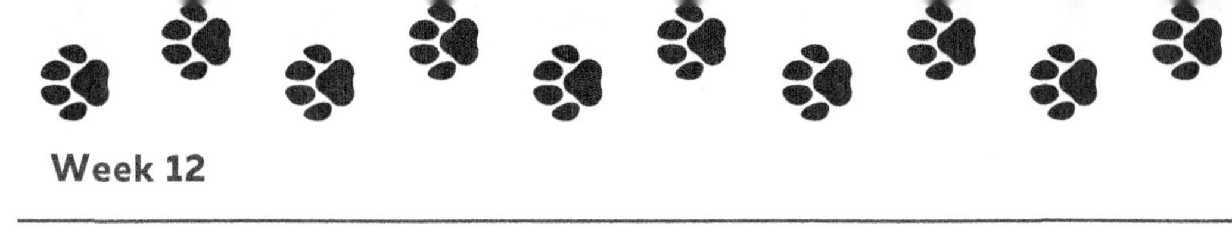

## Week 12

### 21 | Monday

### 22 | Tuesday

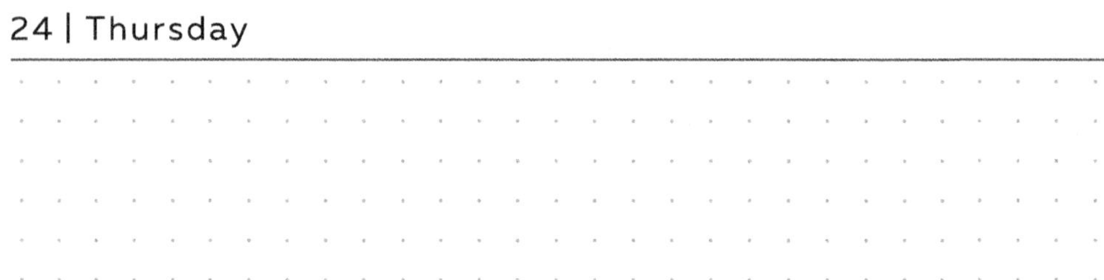

### 23 | Wednesday

### 24 | Thursday

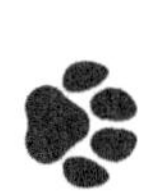
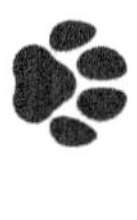
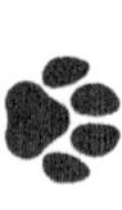
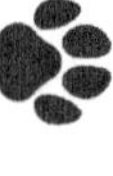
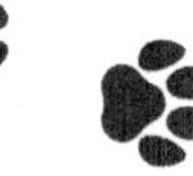

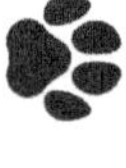
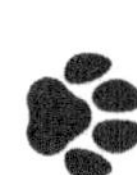
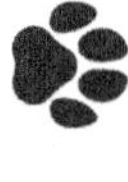
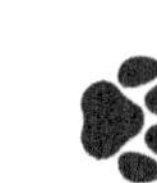
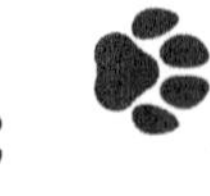

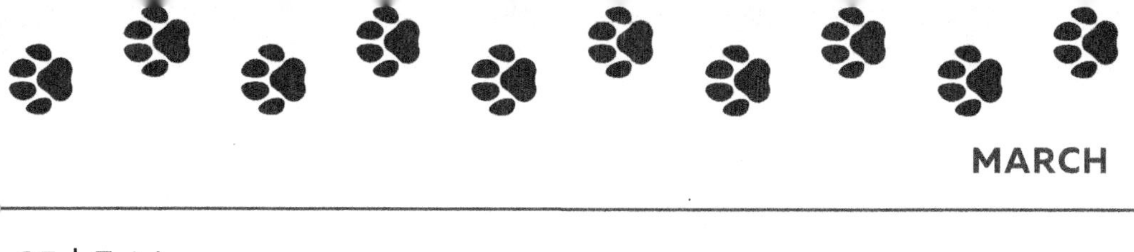

MARCH

25 | Friday

26 | Saturday

27 | Sunday

Notes

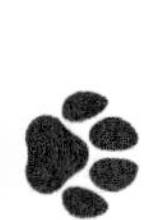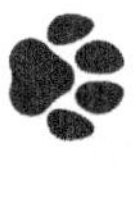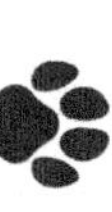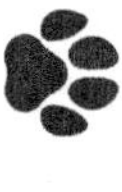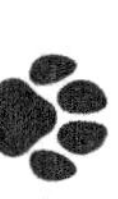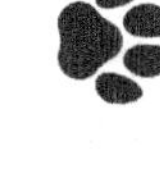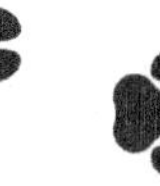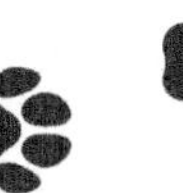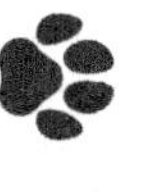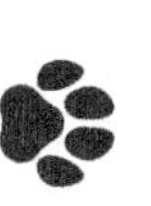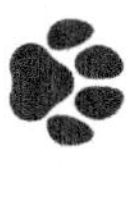

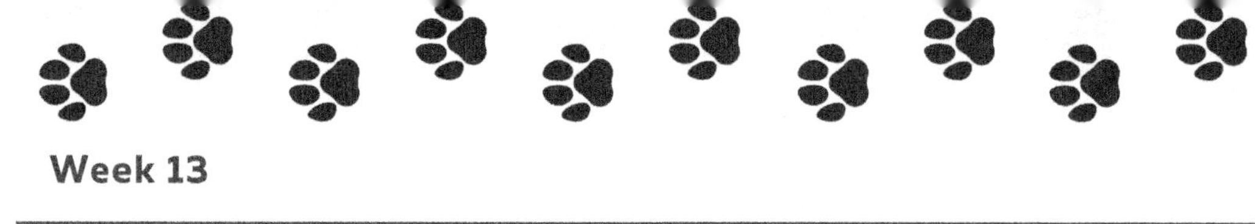

## Week 13

### 28 | Monday

### 29 | Tuesday

### 30 | Wednesday

### 31 | Thursday

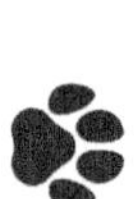
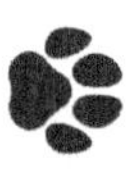
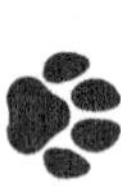
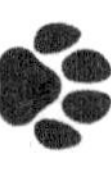

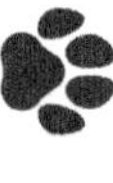
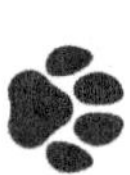
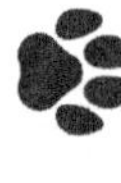
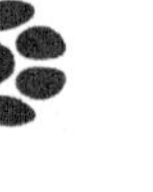
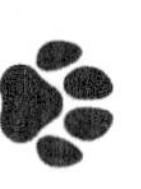
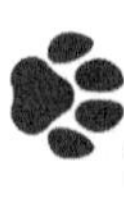

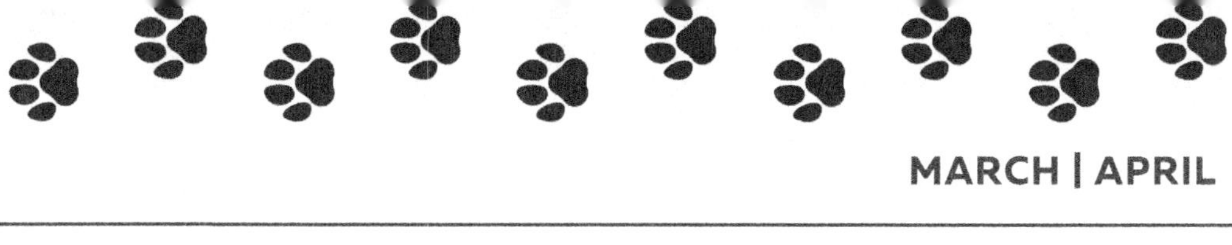



1 | Friday

2 | Saturday

3 | Sunday

Notes

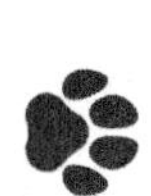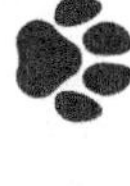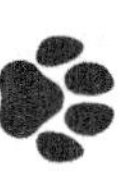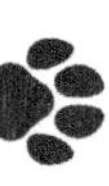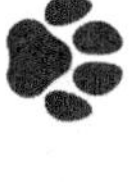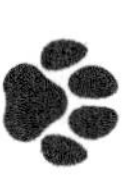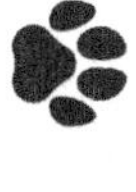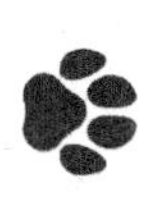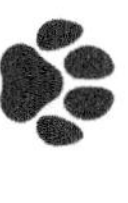

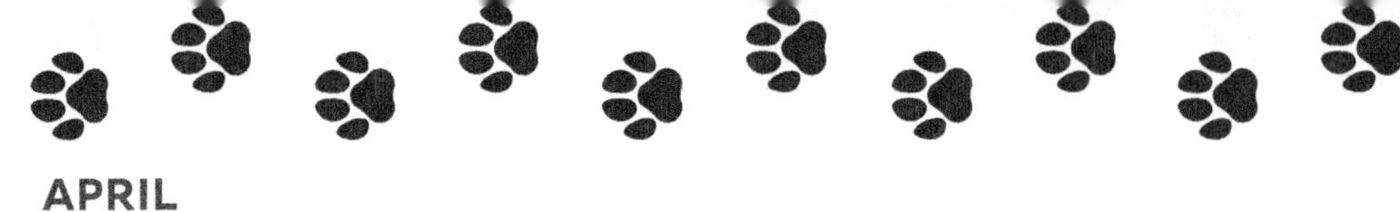

## APRIL

| Monday | Tuesday | Wednesday | Thursday |
| --- | --- | --- | --- |
| | | | |
| 4 | 5 | 6 | 7 |
| 11 | 12 | 13 | 14 |
| 18 Easter Monday | 19 | 20 | 21 |
| 25 St. George's Day | 26 | 27 | 28 |

2022

| Friday | Saturday | Sunday |
| --- | --- | --- |
| 1 | 2 | 3 |
| 8 | 9 | 10 |
| 15 Good Friday | 16 | 17 Easter Sunday |
| 22 | 23 | 24 |
| 29 | 30 | |

Goals

To Do

Reminder

Notes

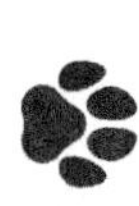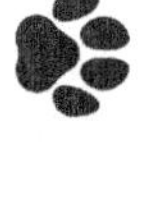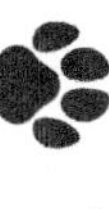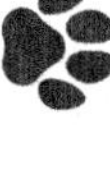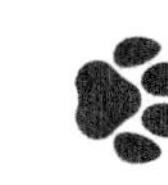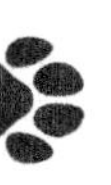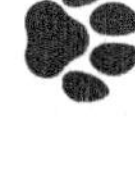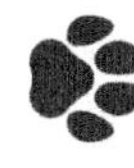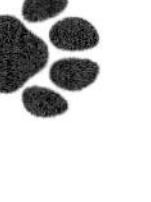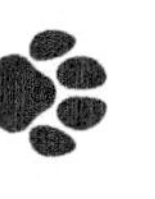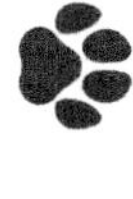

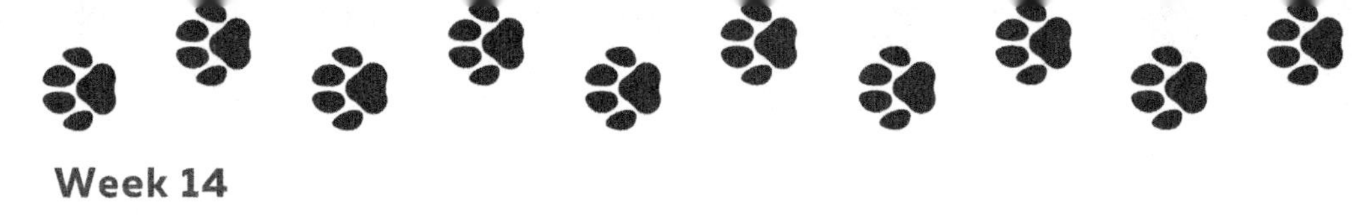

**Week 14**

4 | Monday

5 | Tuesday

6 | Wednesday

7 | Thursday

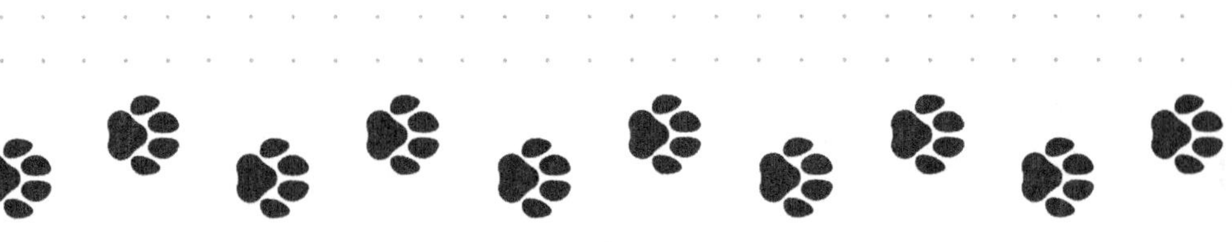

8 | Friday

9 | Saturday

10 | Sunday

Notes

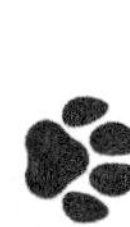
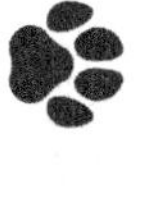
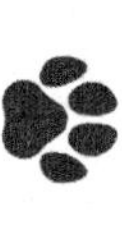
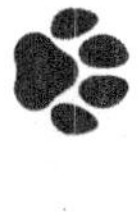
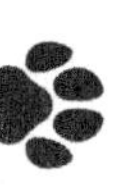
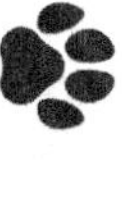
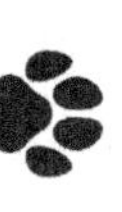
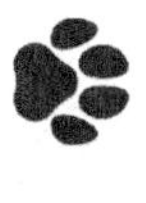
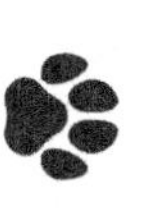
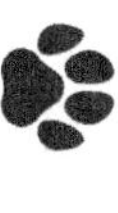

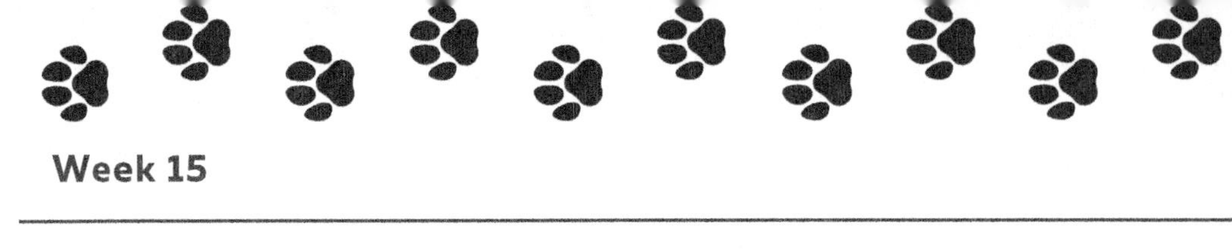

## Week 15

11 | Monday

12 | Tuesday

13 | Wednesday

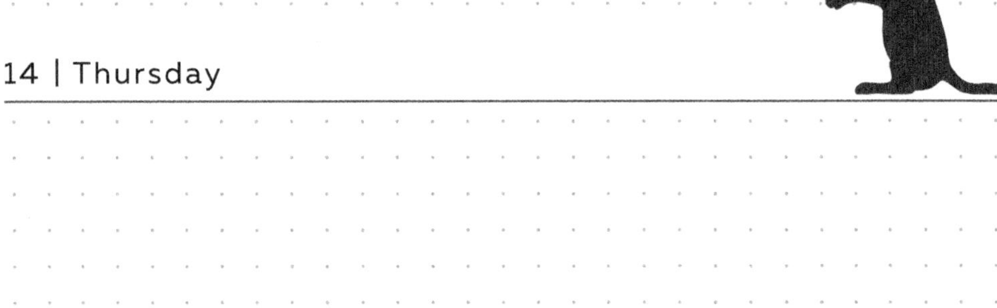

14 | Thursday

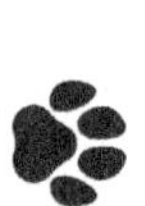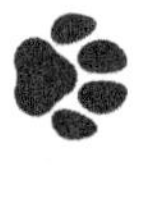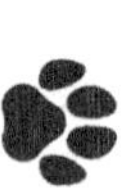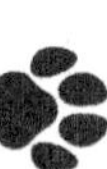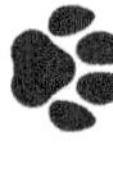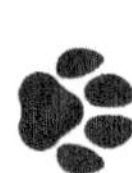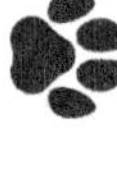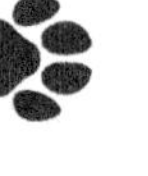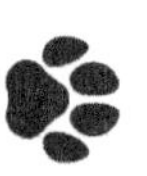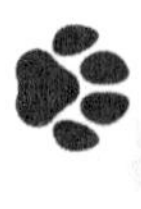

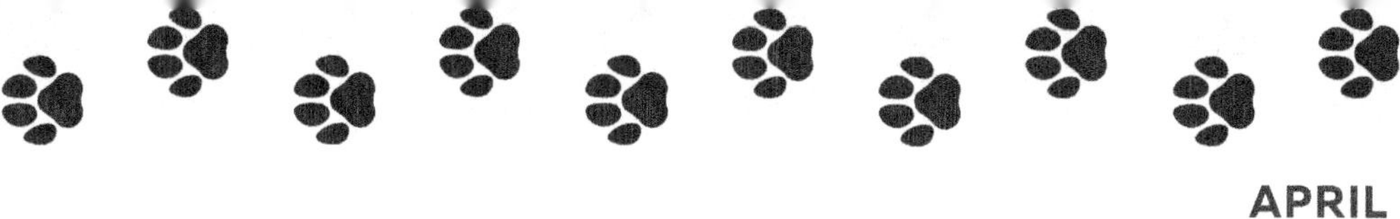



15 | Friday — Good Friday

16 | Saturday

17 | Sunday — Easter Sunday

Notes

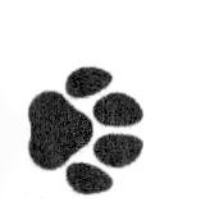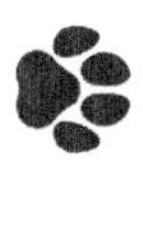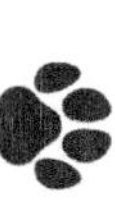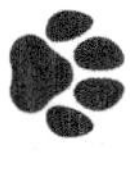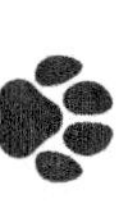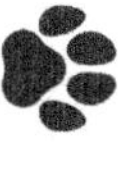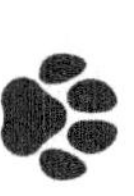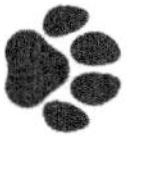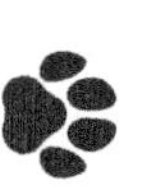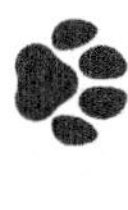

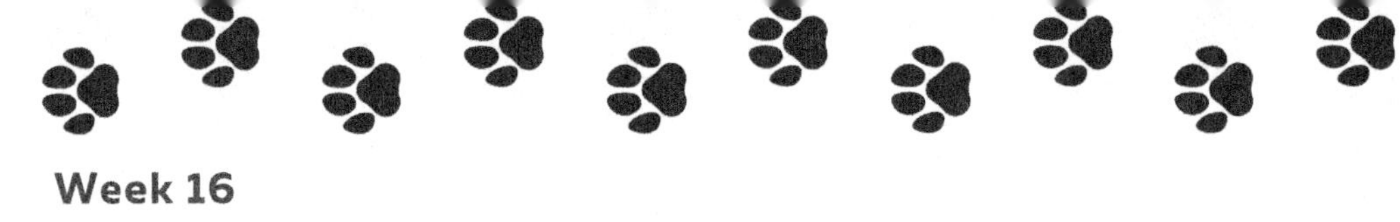

## Week 16

18 | Monday Easter Monday

19 | Tuesday

20 | Wednesday

21 | Thursday

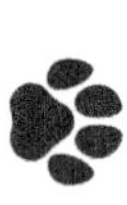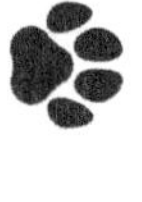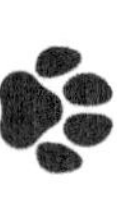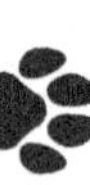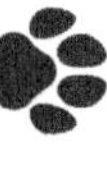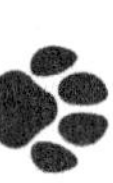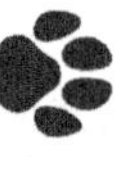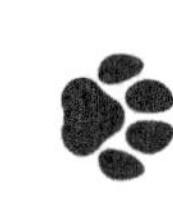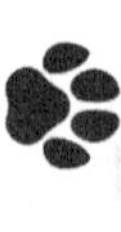

22 | Friday

23 | Saturday

24 | Sunday

Notes

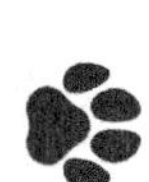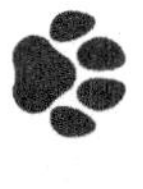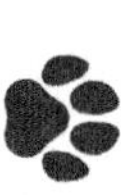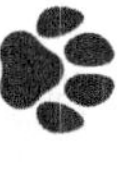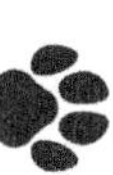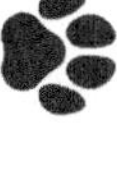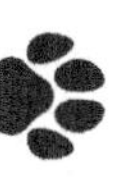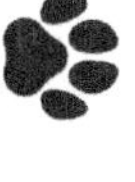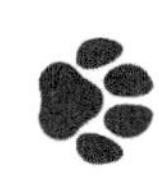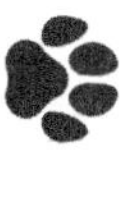

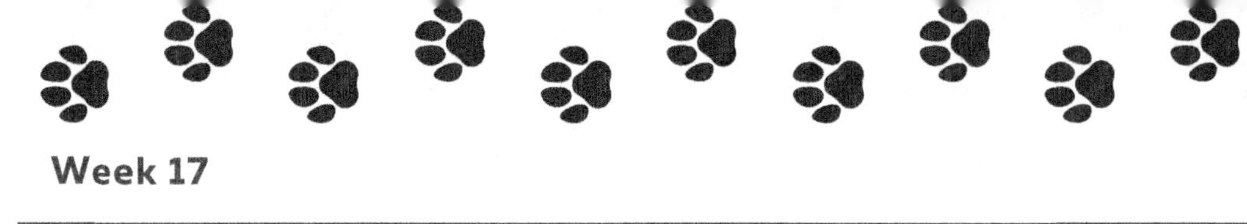

## Week 17

### 25 | Monday

St. George's Day

### 26 | Tuesday

### 27 | Wednesday

### 28 | Thursday

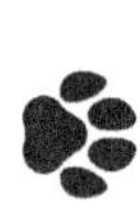
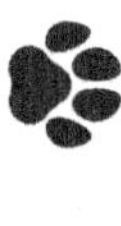
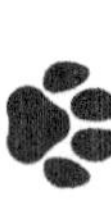

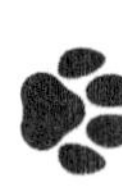

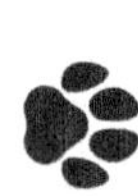
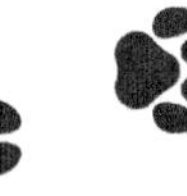
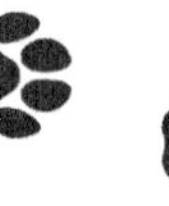
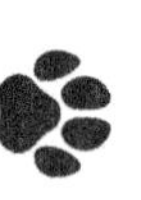
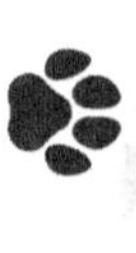

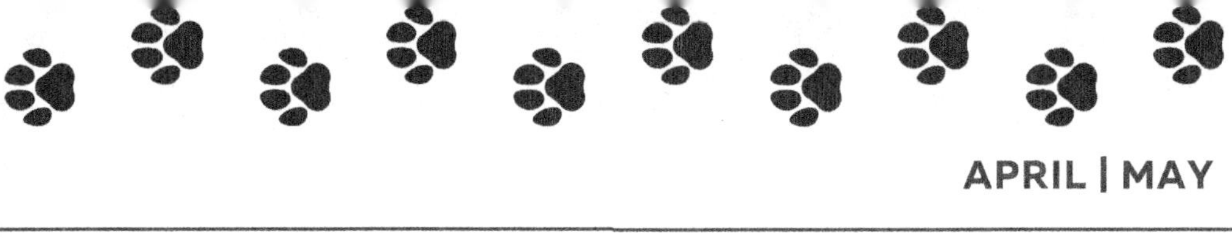



29 | Friday

30 | Saturday

1 | Sunday

Notes

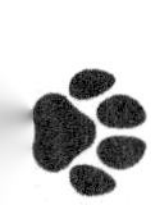
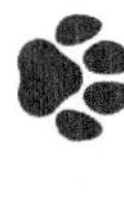
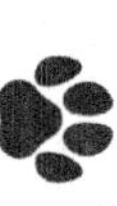
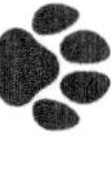
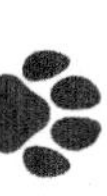
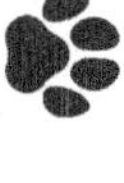
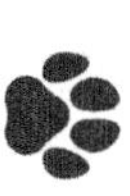
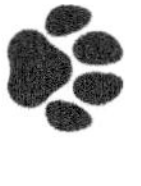
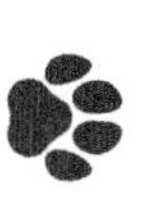
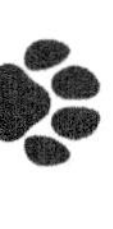

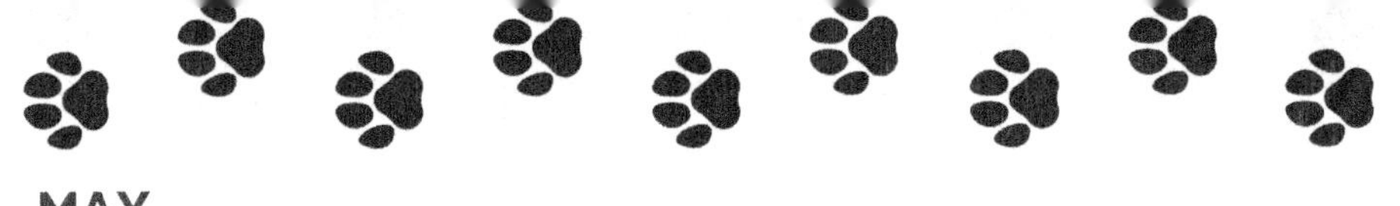

# MAY

| Monday | Tuesday | Wednesday | Thursday |
|---|---|---|---|
| | | | |
| 2 Early May Bank Holiday | 3 | 4 | 5 |
| 9 | 10 | 11 | 12 |
| 16 | 17 | 18 | 19 |
| 23 | 24 | 25 | 26 |
| 30 | 31 | | |

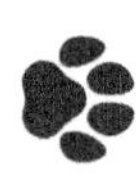
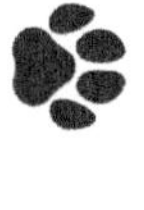
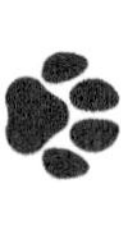

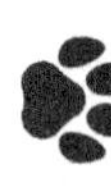
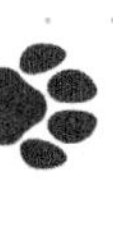
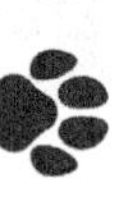
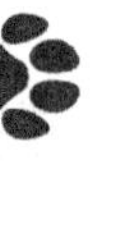
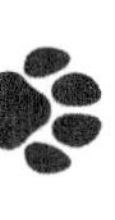
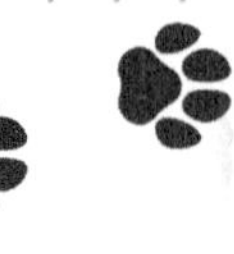

2022

| Friday | Saturday | Sunday |
|---|---|---|
| | | 1 |
| 6 | 7 | 8 Mother's Day |
| 13 | 14 | 15 |
| 20 | 21 | 22 |
| 27 | 28 | 29 |

Goals

To Do

Reminder

Notes

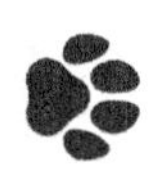
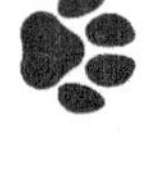
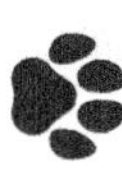
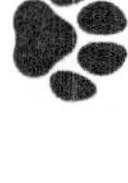

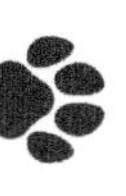
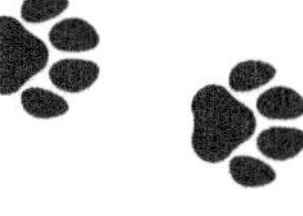
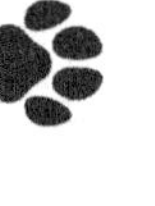
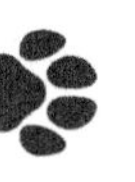
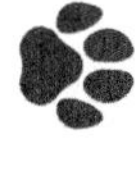

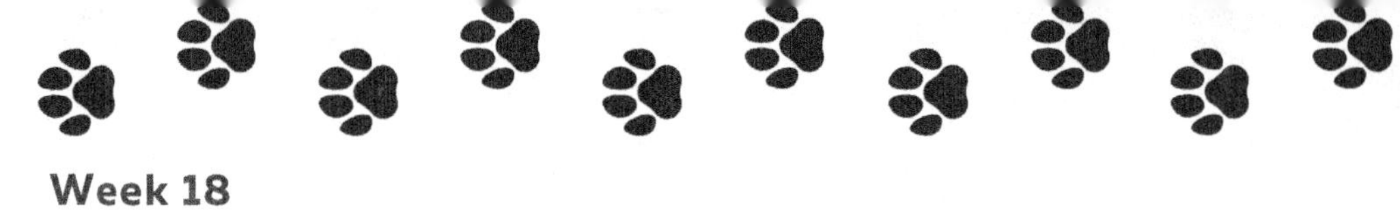

## Week 18

### 2 | Monday

Early May Bank Holiday

### 3 | Tuesday

### 4 | Wednesday

### 5 | Thursday

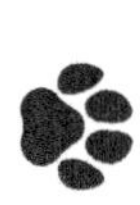 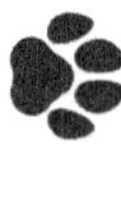 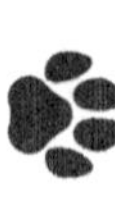   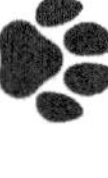 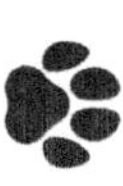 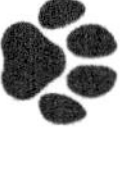 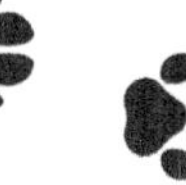 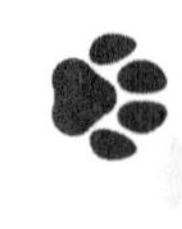

6 | Friday

7 | Saturday

8 | Sunday Mother's Day

Notes

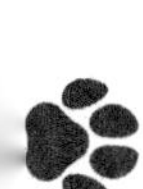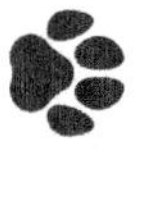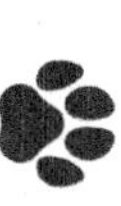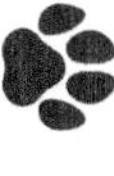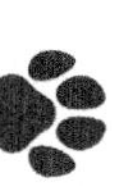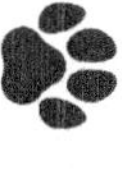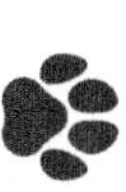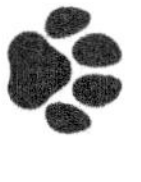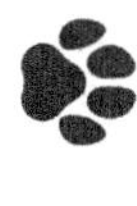

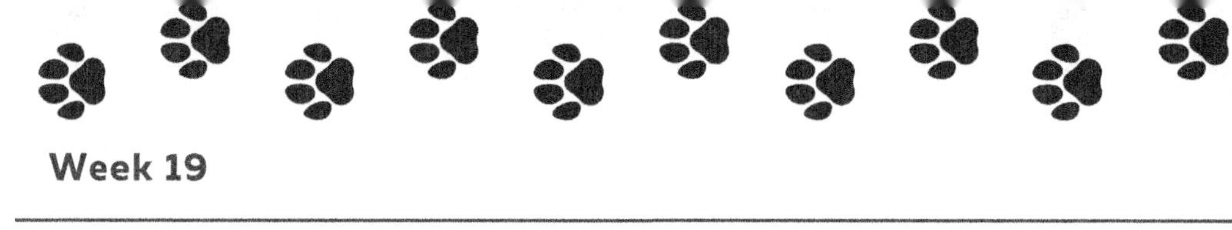

## Week 19

9 | Monday

10 | Tuesday

11 | Wednesday

12 | Thursday

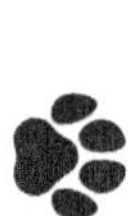
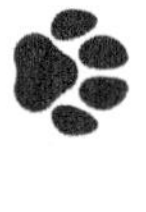
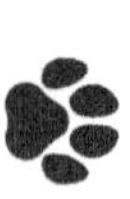

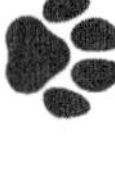
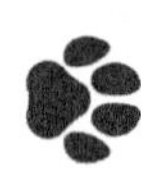
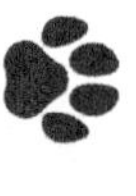
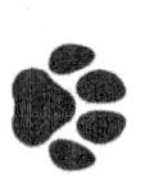
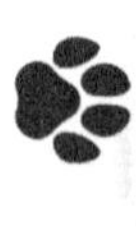

13 | Friday

14 | Saturday

15 | Sunday

Notes

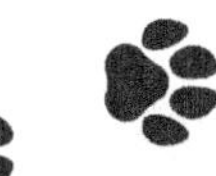
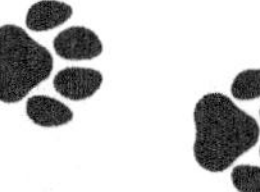
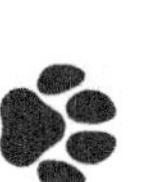
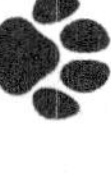

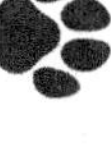
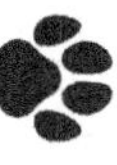
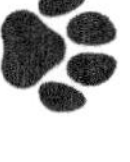
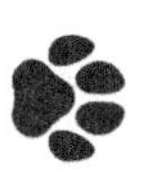
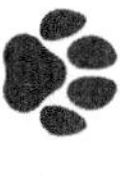

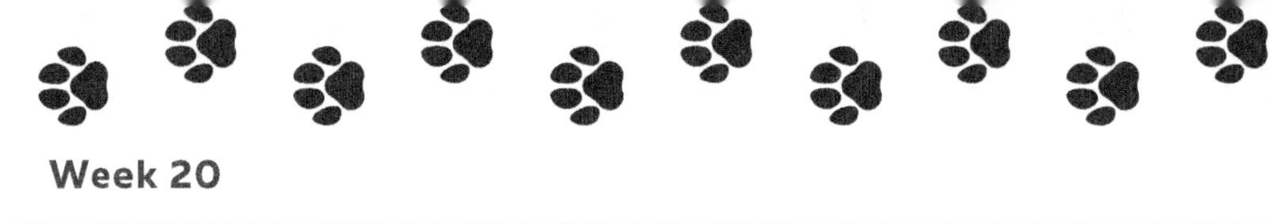

## Week 20

### 16 | Monday

### 17 | Tuesday

### 18 | Wednesday

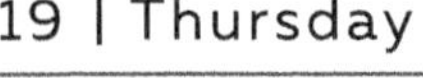

### 19 | Thursday

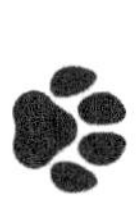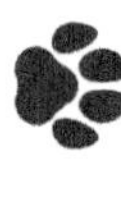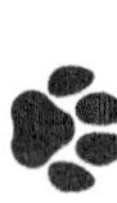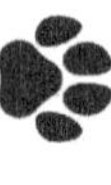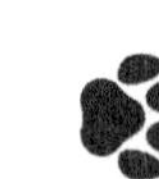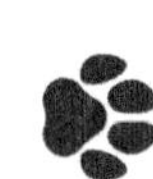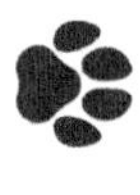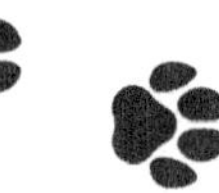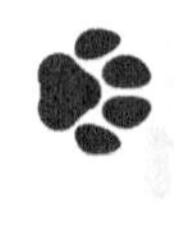

MAY

20 | Friday

21 | Saturday

22 | Sunday

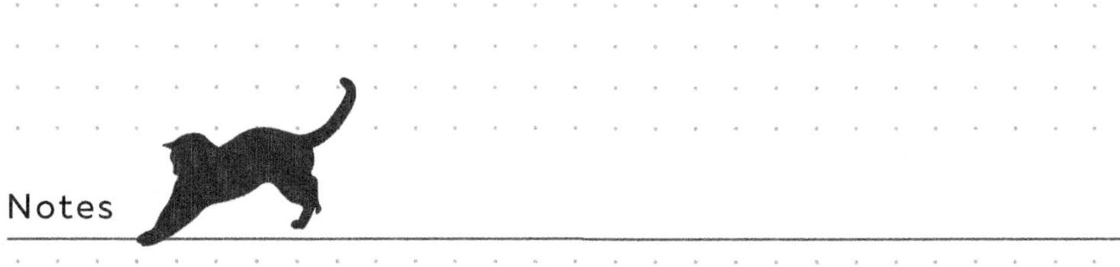

Notes

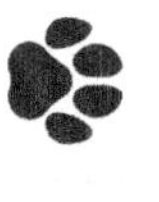
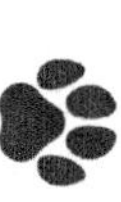
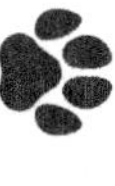
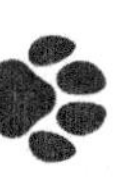
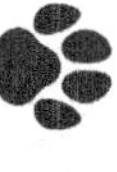
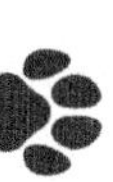
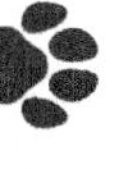
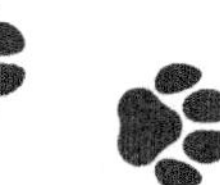
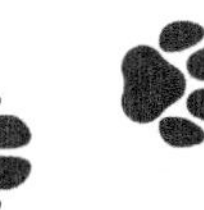

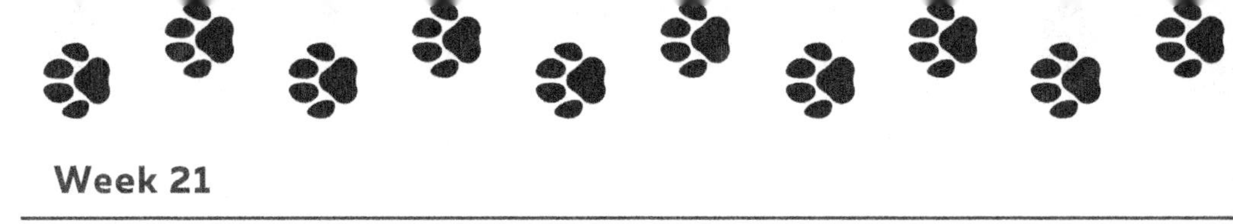

## Week 21

### 23 | Monday

### 24 | Tuesday

### 25 | Wednesday

### 26 | Thursday

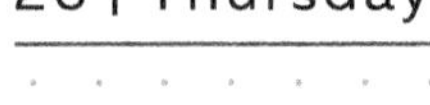

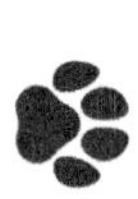
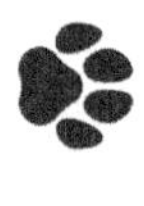
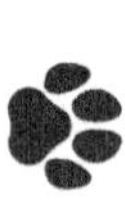
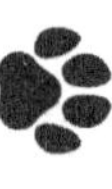

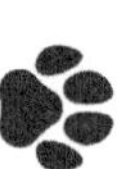
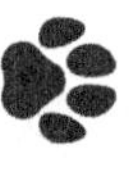
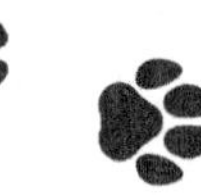
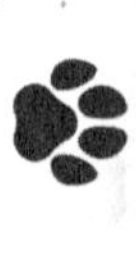

27 | Friday

28 | Saturday

29 | Sunday

Notes

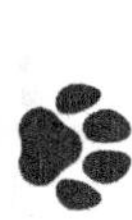 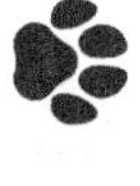 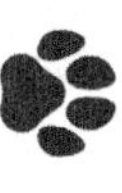 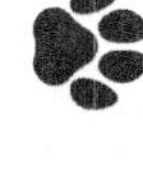 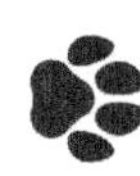  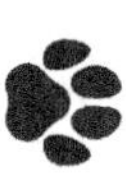 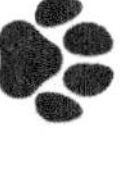 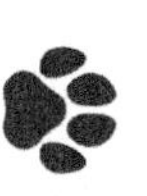 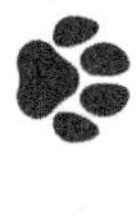

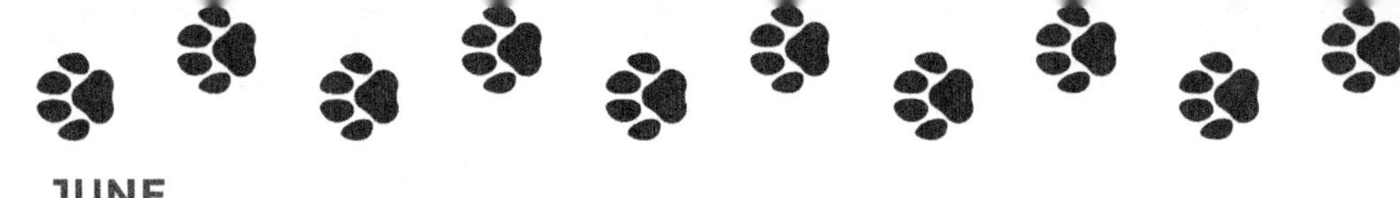

# JUNE

| Monday | Tuesday | Wednesday | Thursday |
|---|---|---|---|
| | | 1 | 2 Spring Bank Holiday |
| 6 | 7 | 8 | 9 |
| 13 | 14 | 15 | 16 |
| 20 | 21 | 22 | 23 |
| 27 | 28 | 29 | 30 |

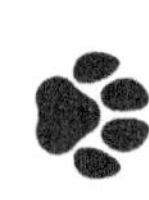

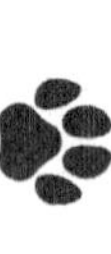

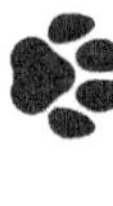
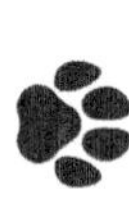
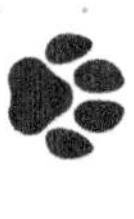
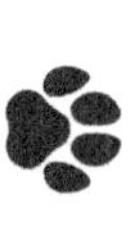
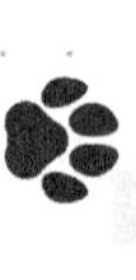

| Friday | Saturday | Sunday |
| --- | --- | --- |
| 3 Queen's Platinum Jubilee | 4 | 5 |
| 10 | 11 Queen's Birthday | 12 |
| 17 | 18 | 19 Father's Day |
| 24 | 25 | 26 |

## Goals

## To Do

## Reminder

## Notes

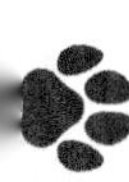
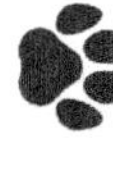
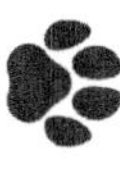
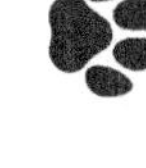
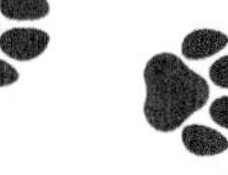
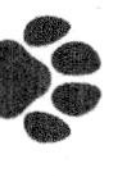
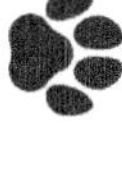
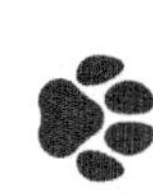
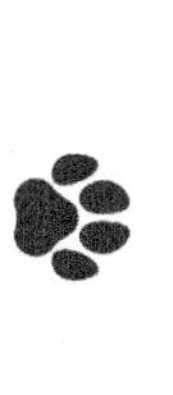
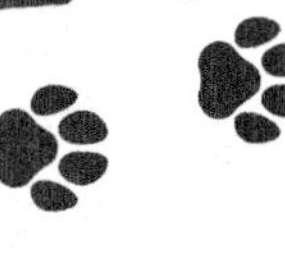

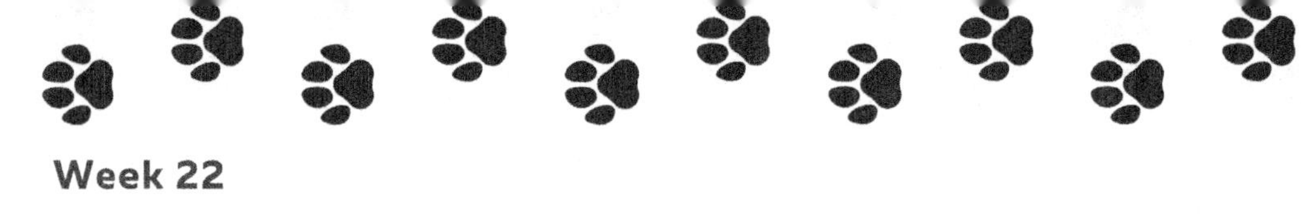

## Week 22

30 | Monday

31 | Tuesday

1 | Wednesday

2 | Thursday

Spring Bank Holiday

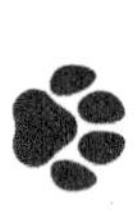
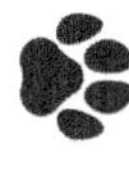
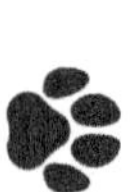
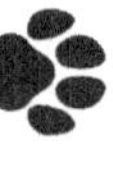

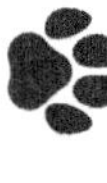
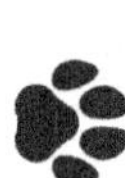
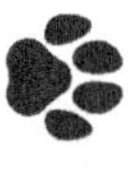
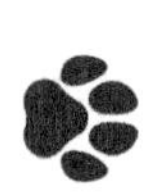
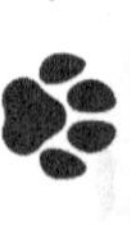

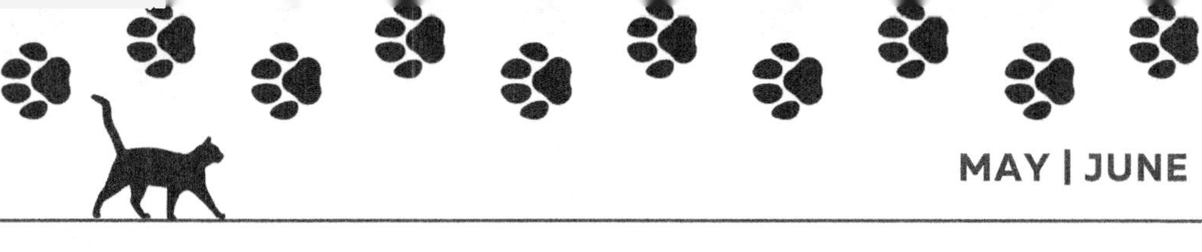



3 | Friday Queen's Platinum Jubilee

4 | Saturday

5 | Sunday

Notes

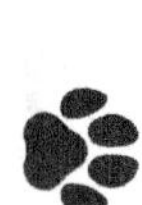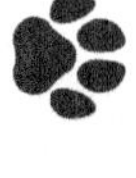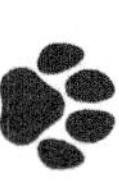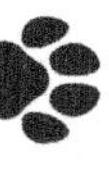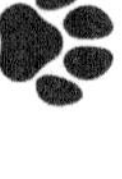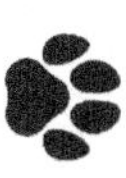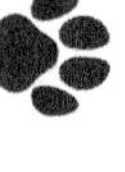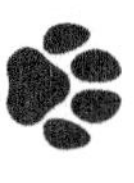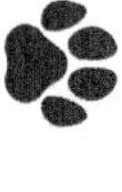

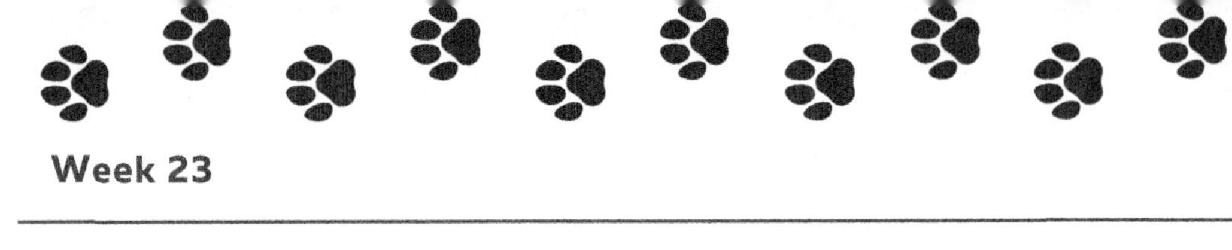

## Week 23

### 6 | Monday

### 7 | Tuesday

### 8 | Wednesday

### 9 | Thursday

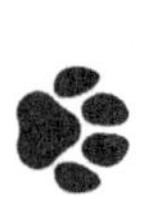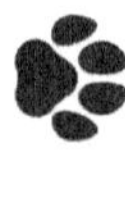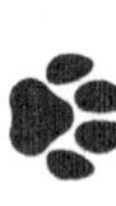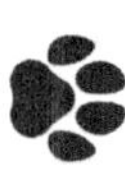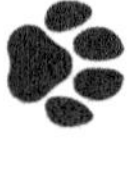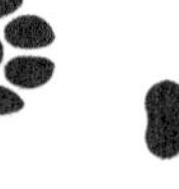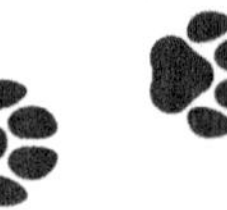

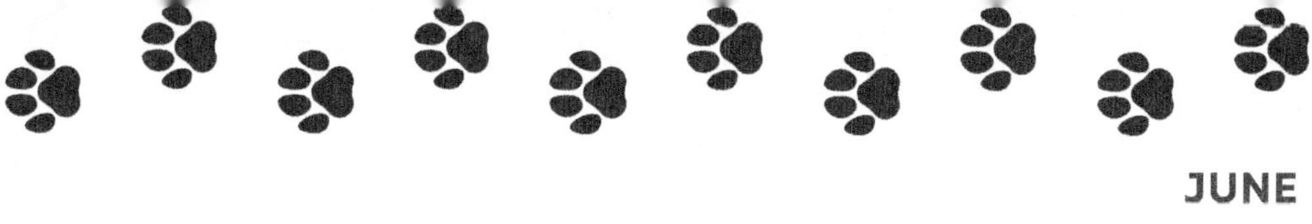



## 10 | Friday

## 11 | Saturday

Queen's Birthday

## 12 | Sunday

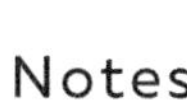

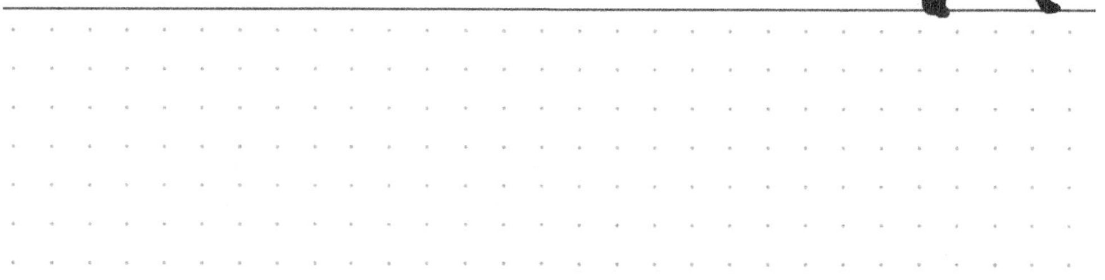

## Notes

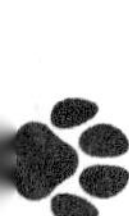
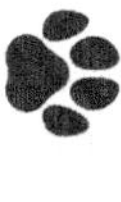
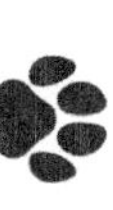
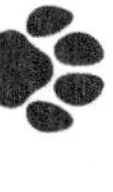
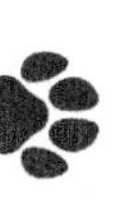
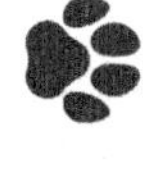
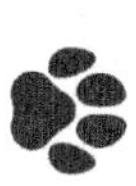
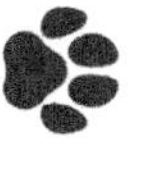
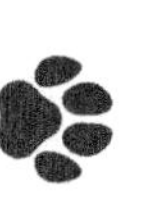
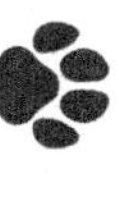

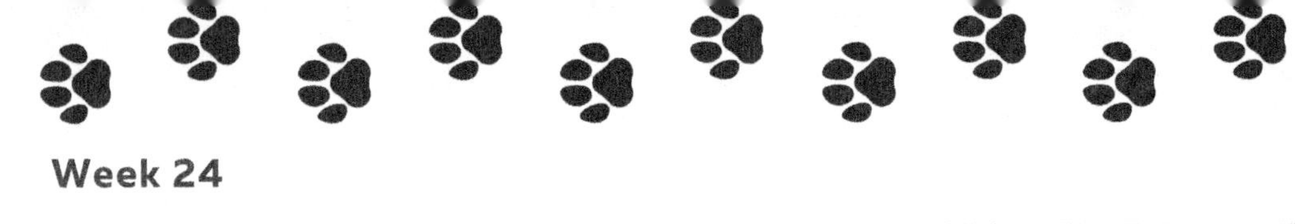

## Week 24

13 | Monday

14 | Tuesday

15 | Wednesday

16 | Thursday

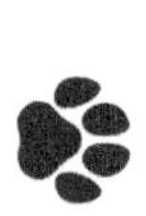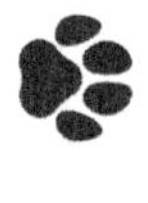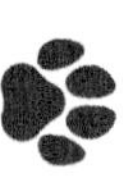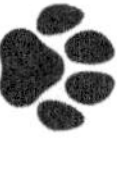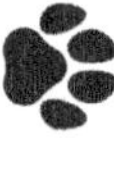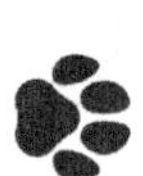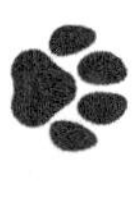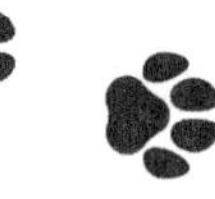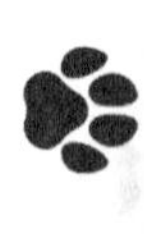

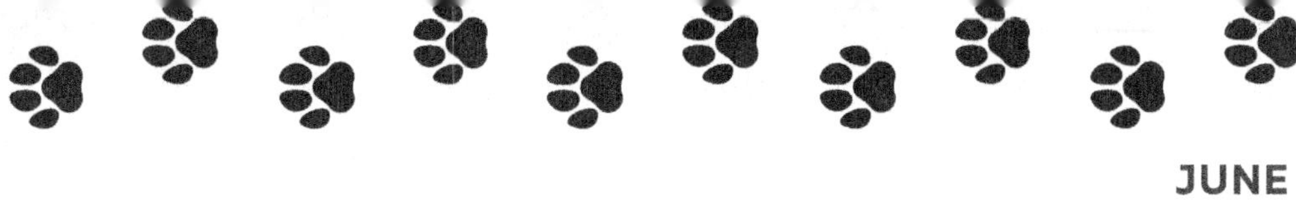



17 | Friday

18 | Saturday

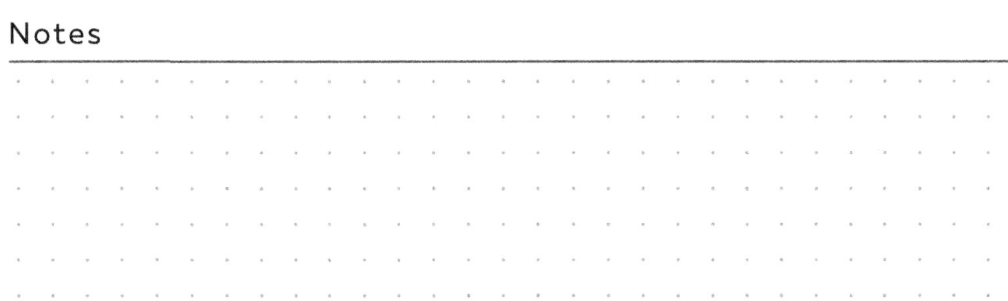

19 | Sunday

Father's Day

Notes

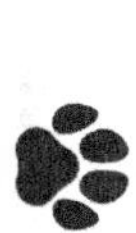
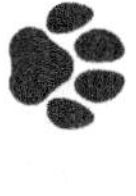
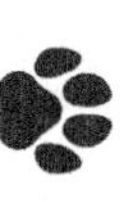

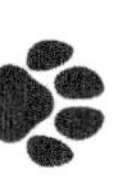
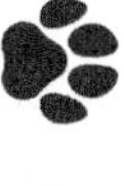
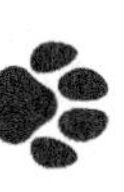
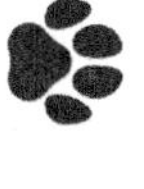
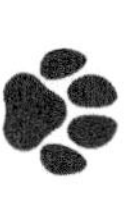
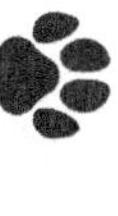

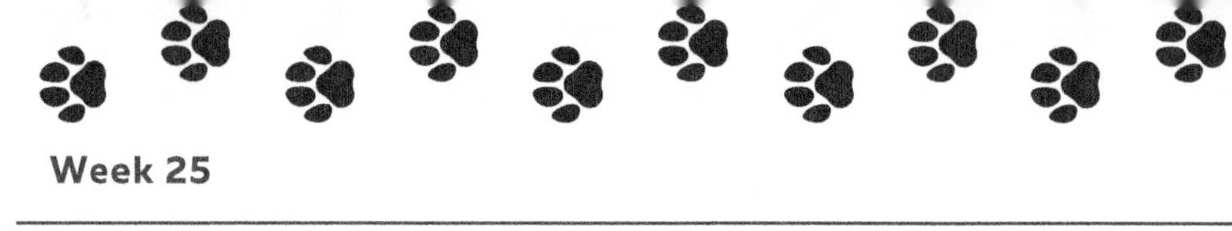

## Week 25

20 | Monday

21 | Tuesday

22 | Wednesday

23 | Thursday

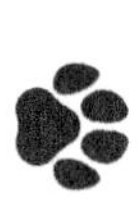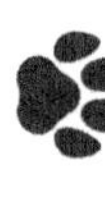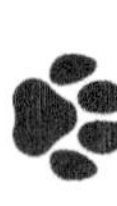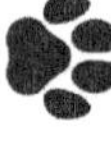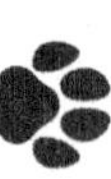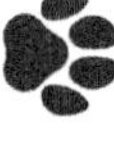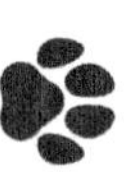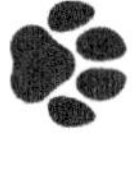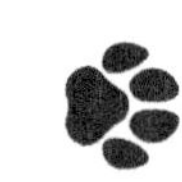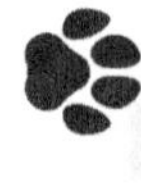

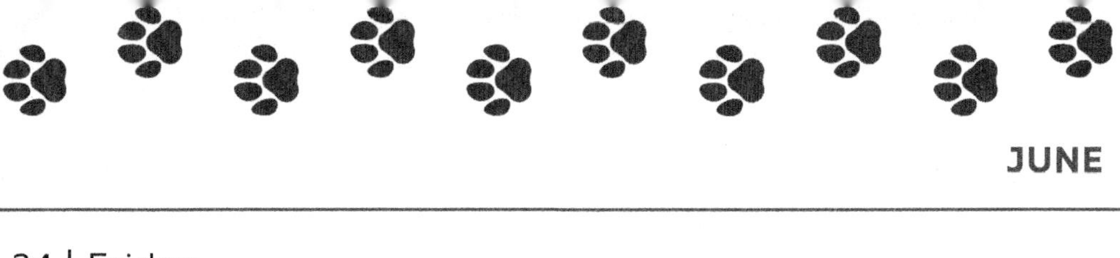



24 | Friday

25 | Saturday

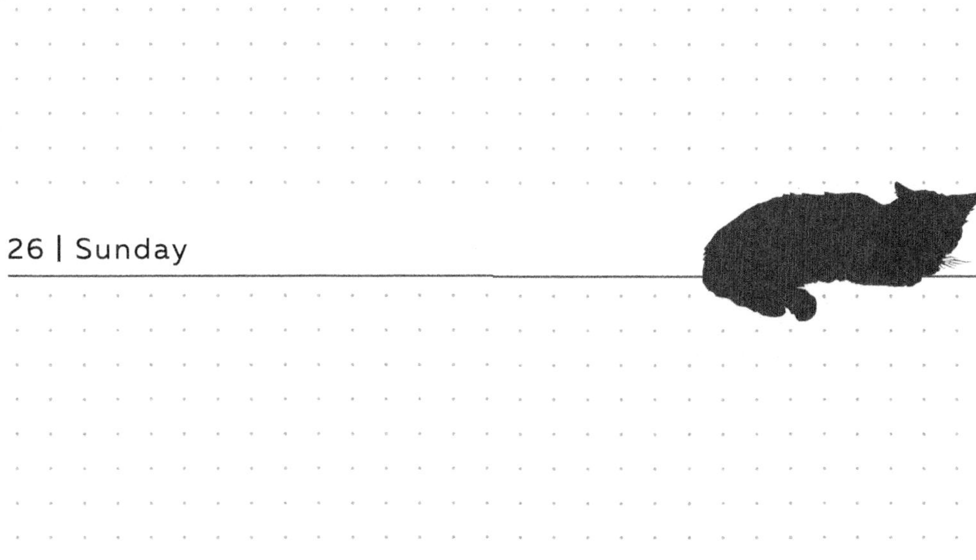

26 | Sunday

Notes

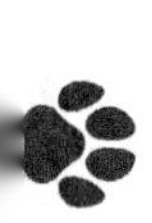

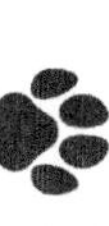
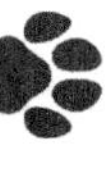
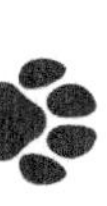
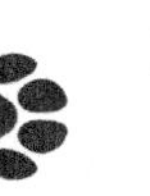

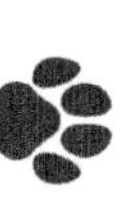
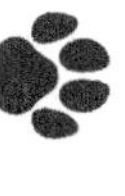
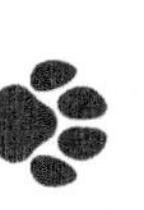
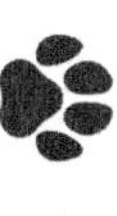

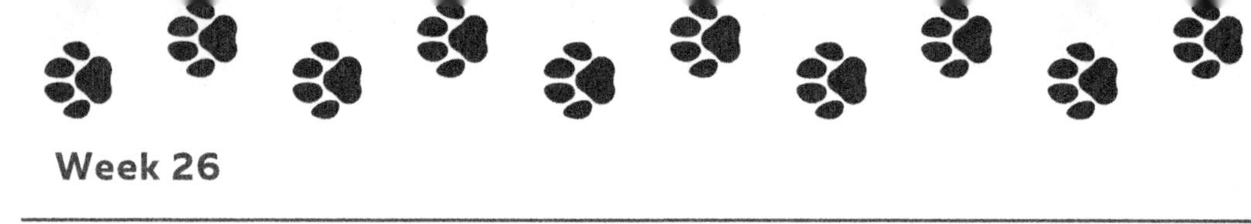

## Week 26

27 | Monday

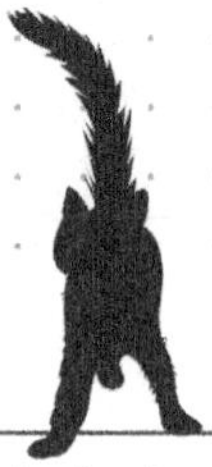

28 | Tuesday

29 | Wednesday

30 | Thursday

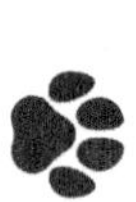 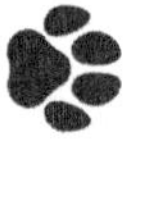 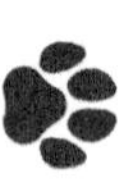  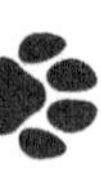 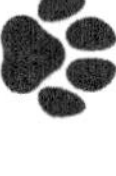 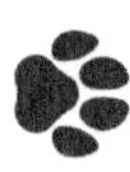 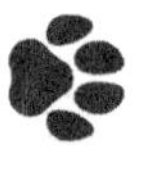 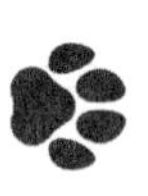 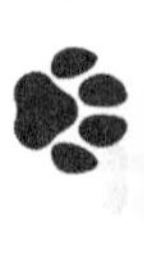

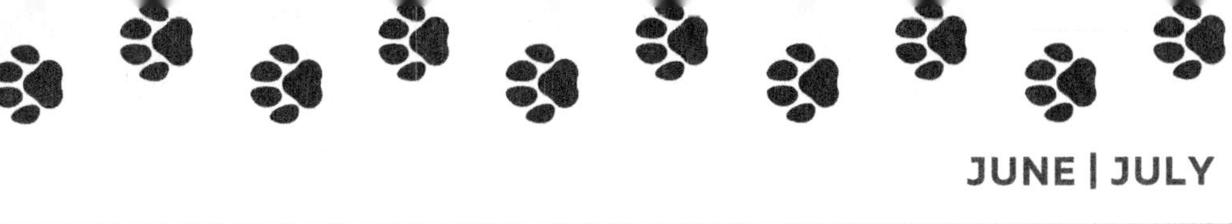



1 | Friday

2 | Saturday

3 | Sunday

Notes

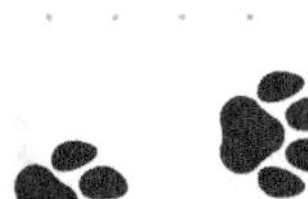
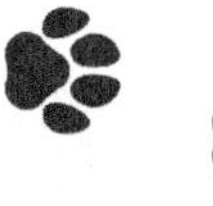
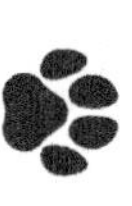

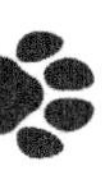

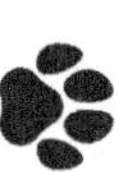
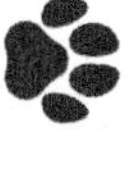
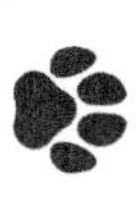
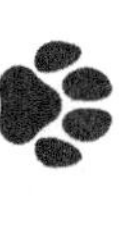

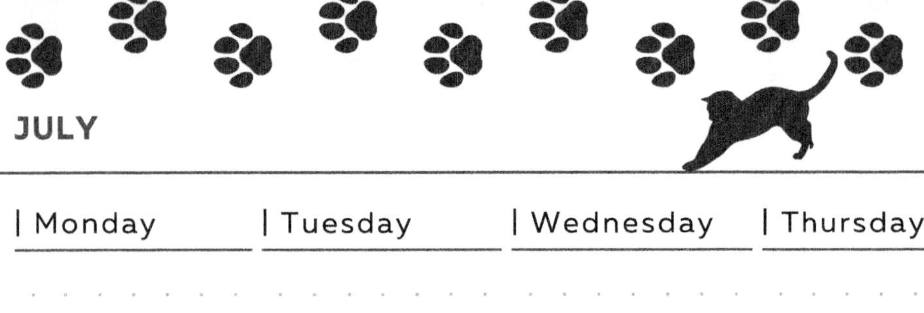

## JULY

| Monday | Tuesday | Wednesday | Thursday |
|---|---|---|---|
| | | | |
| 4 | 5 | 6 | 7 |
| 11 | 12 | 13 | 14 |
| 18 | 19 | 20 | 21 |
| 25 | 26 | 27 | 28 |

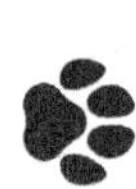
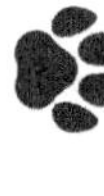
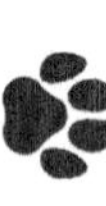
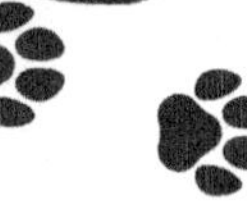
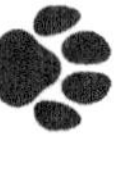
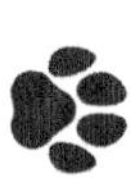
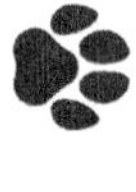
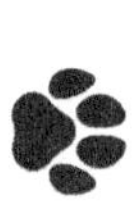
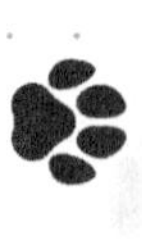

2022

| Friday | Saturday | Sunday |
|---|---|---|
| 1 | 2 | 3 |
| 8 | 9 | 10 |
| 15 | 16 | 17 |
| 22 | 23 | 24 |
| 29 | 30 | 31 |

Goals

To Do

Reminder

Notes

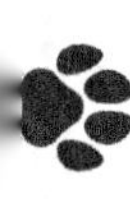

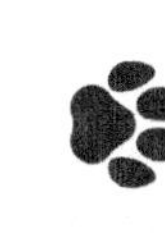
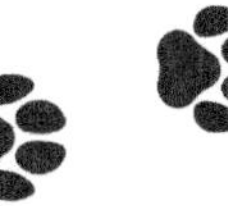
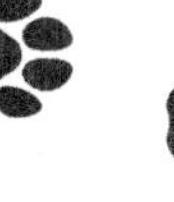

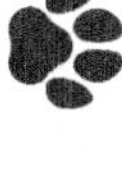
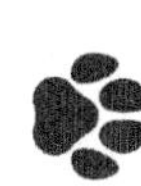
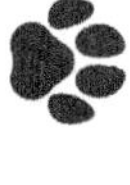
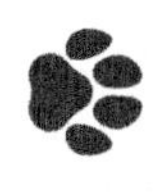
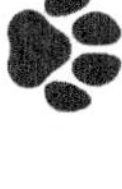

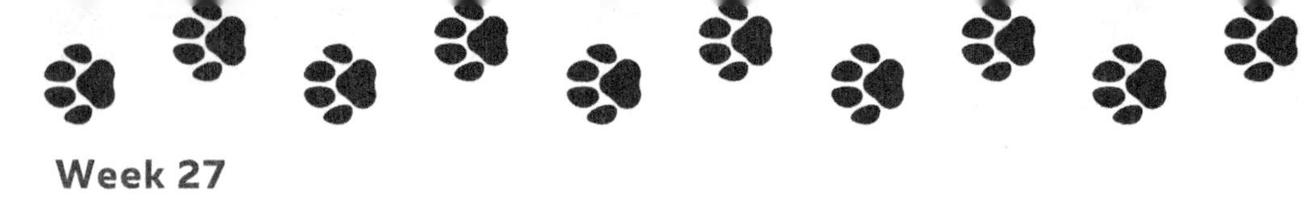

## Week 27

4 | Monday

5 | Tuesday

6 | Wednesday

7 | Thursday

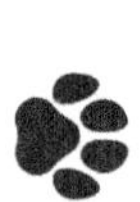 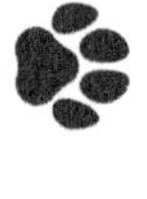 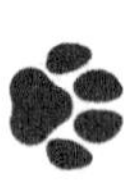 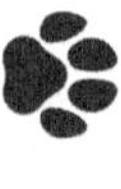 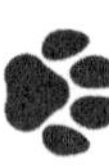 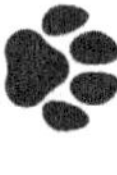 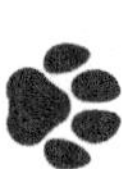 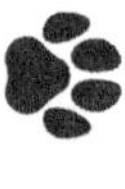 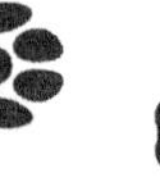 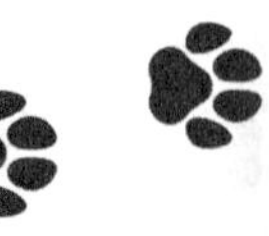

8 | Friday

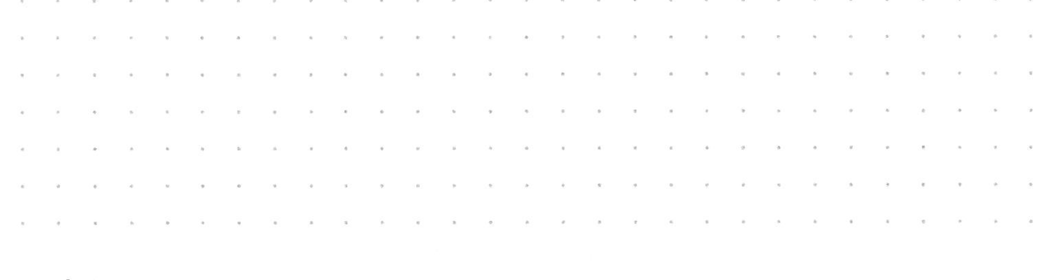

9 | Saturday

10 | Sunday

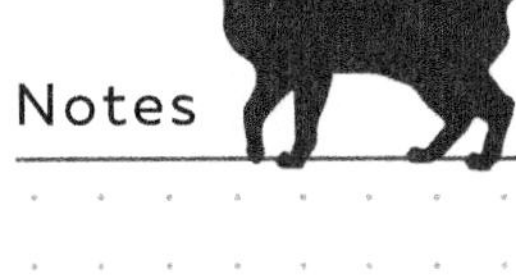

Notes

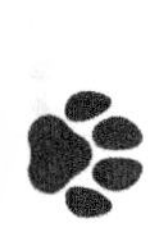
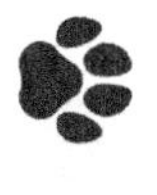
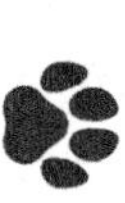
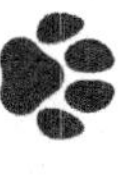
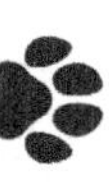
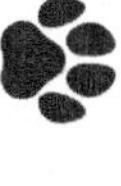
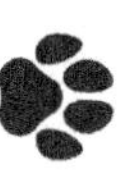
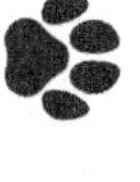
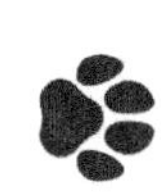
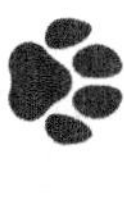

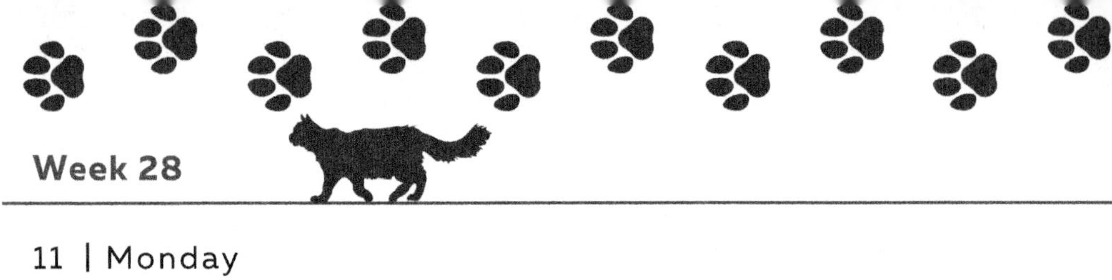

## Week 28

### 11 | Monday

### 12 | Tuesday

### 13 | Wednesday

### 14 | Thursday

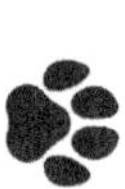
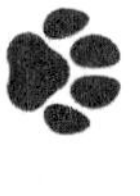
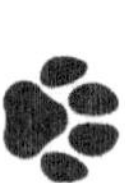

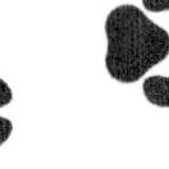
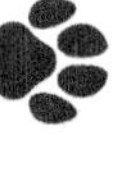
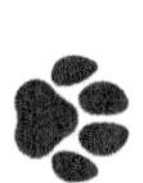
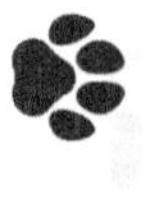

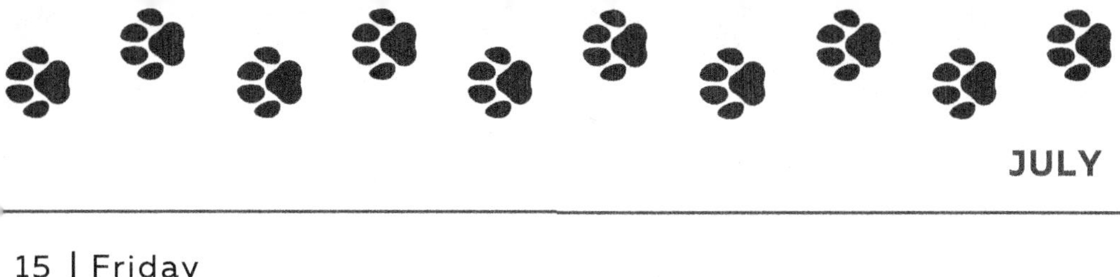



## 15 | Friday

## 16 | Saturday

## 17 | Sunday

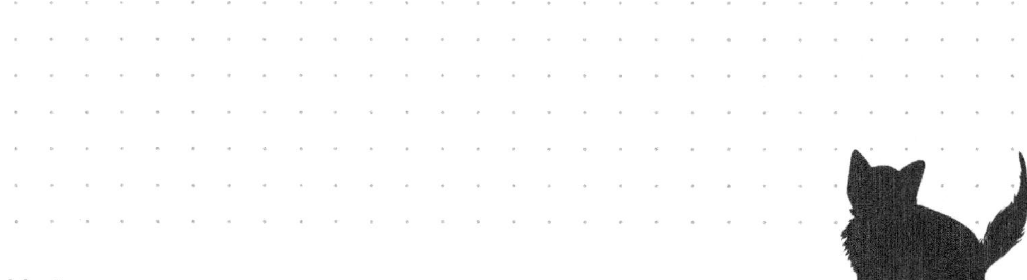

## Notes

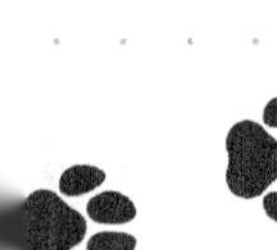
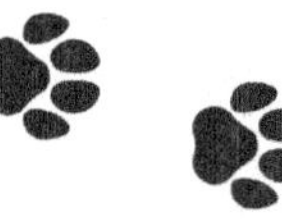
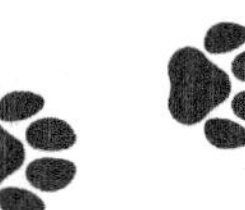

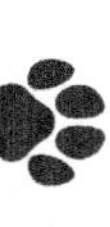
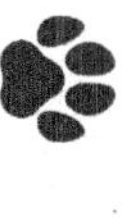
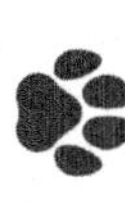
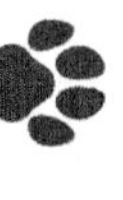

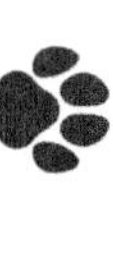

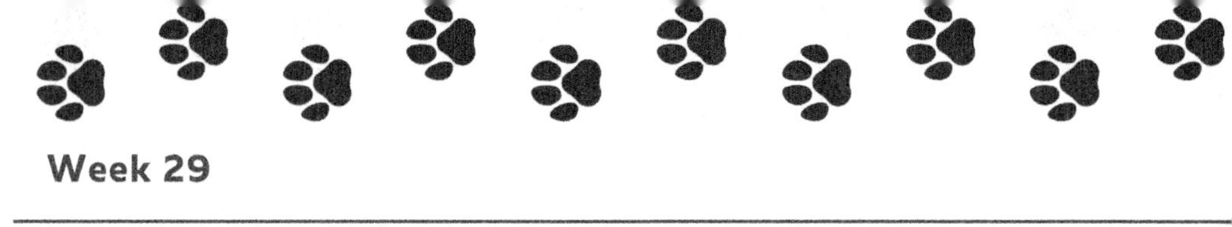

## Week 29

### 18 | Monday

### 19 | Tuesday

### 20 | Wednesday

### 21 | Thursday

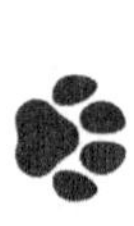
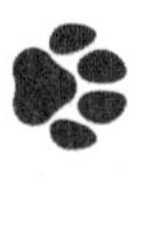
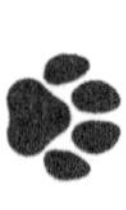

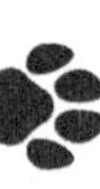

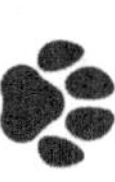
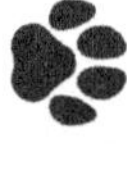
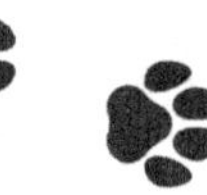
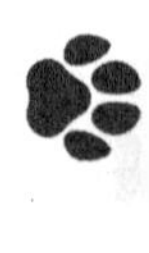

22 | Friday

23 | Saturday

24 | Sunday

Notes

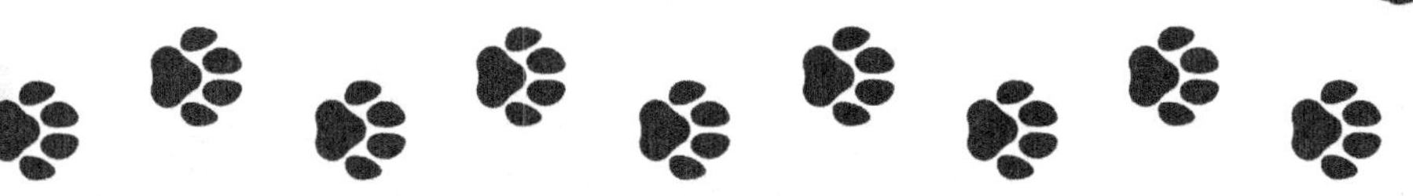

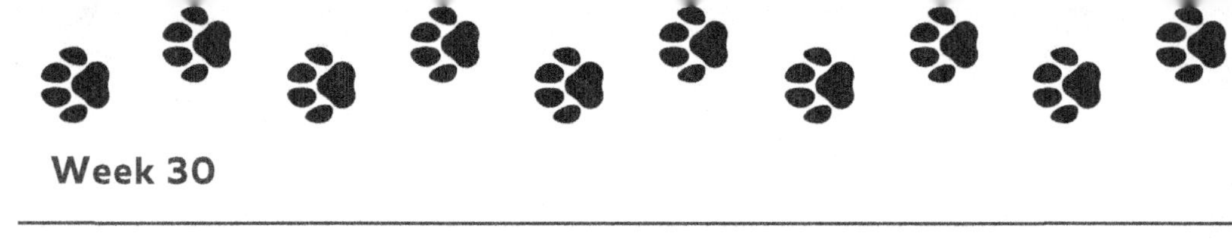

## Week 30

25 | Monday

26 | Tuesday

27 | Wednesday

28 | Thursday

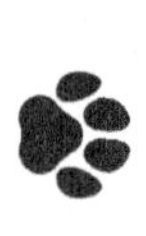
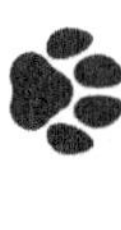
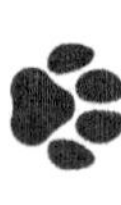
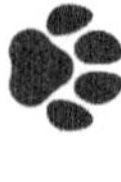
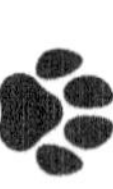
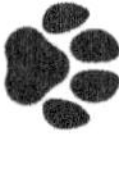
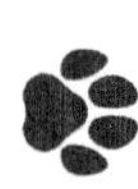
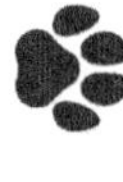

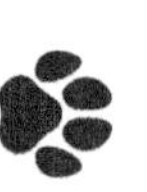
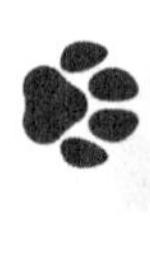

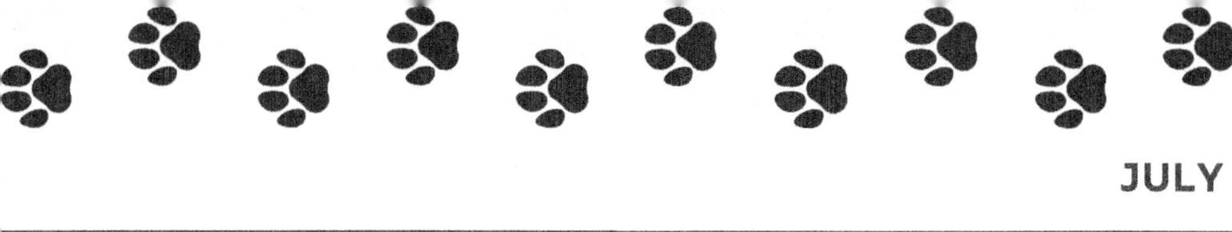



29 | Friday

30 | Saturday

31 | Sunday

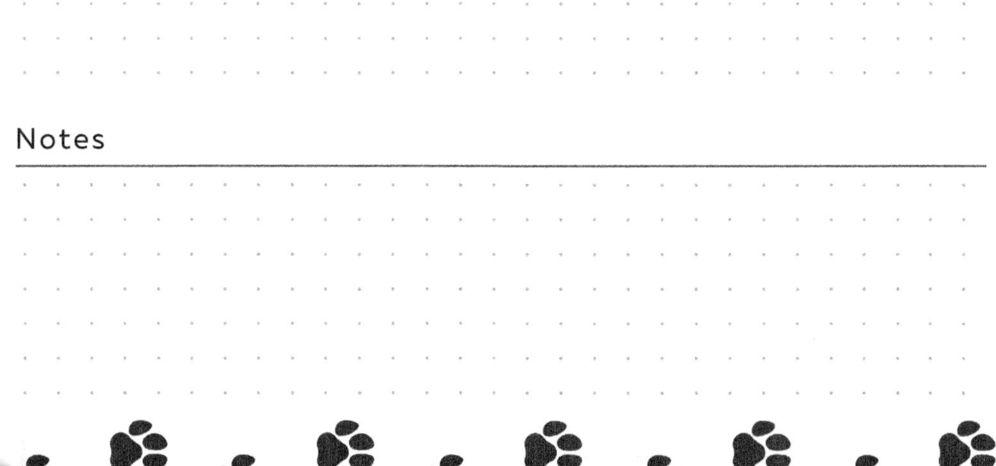

Notes

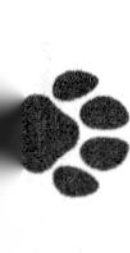
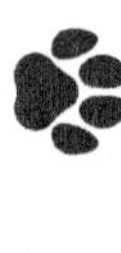
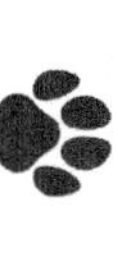
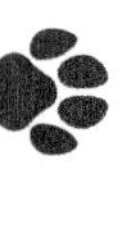
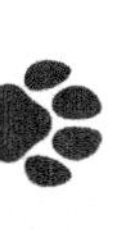
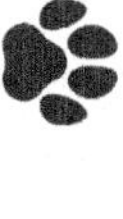
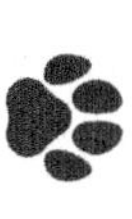
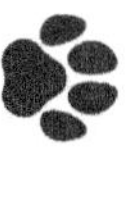
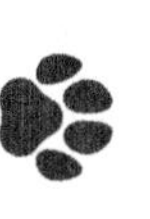
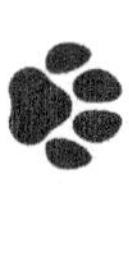

## AUGUST

| Monday | Tuesday | Wednesday | Thursday |
| --- | --- | --- | --- |
| 1 | 2 | 3 | 4 |
| 8 | 9 | 10 | 11 |
| 15 | 16 | 17 | 18 |
| 22 | 23 | 24 | 25 |
| 29 | 30 | 31 | |

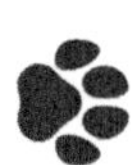

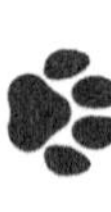

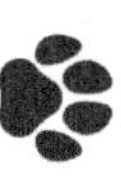
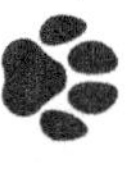
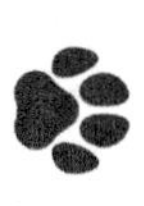

2022

| Friday | Saturday | Sunday |
|---|---|---|
| 5 | 6 | 7 |
| 12 | 13 | 14 |
| 19 | 20 | 21 |
| 26 | 27 | 28 |

Goals

To Do

Reminder

Notes

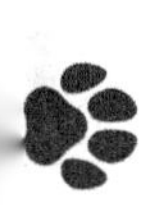
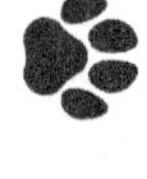
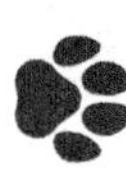
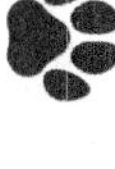
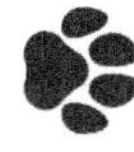
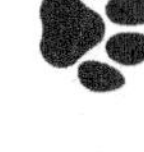
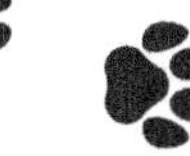
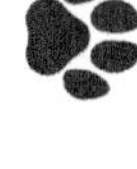
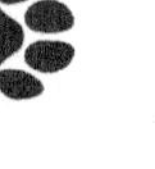
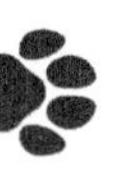
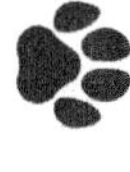

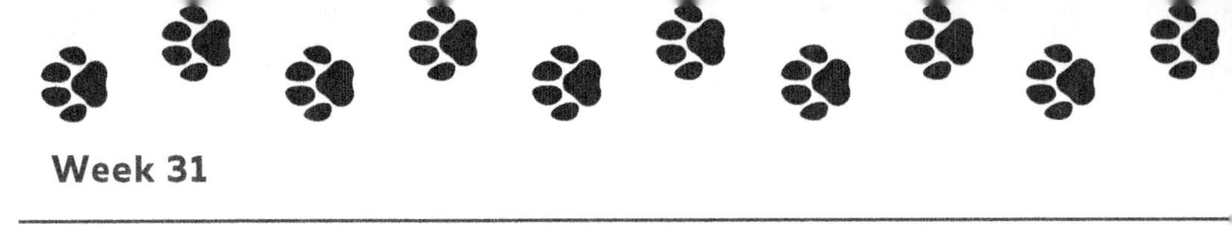

## Week 31

1 | Monday

2 | Tuesday

3 | Wednesday

4 | Thursday

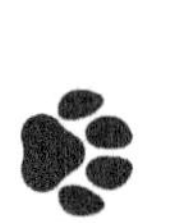
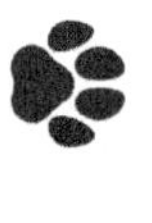
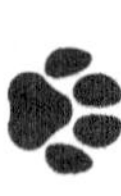

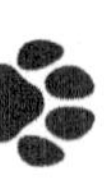
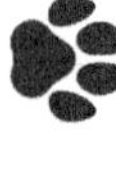
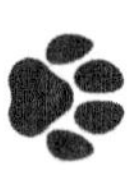
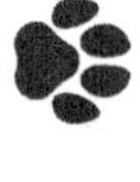
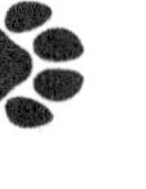
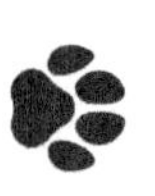
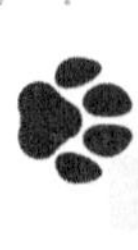

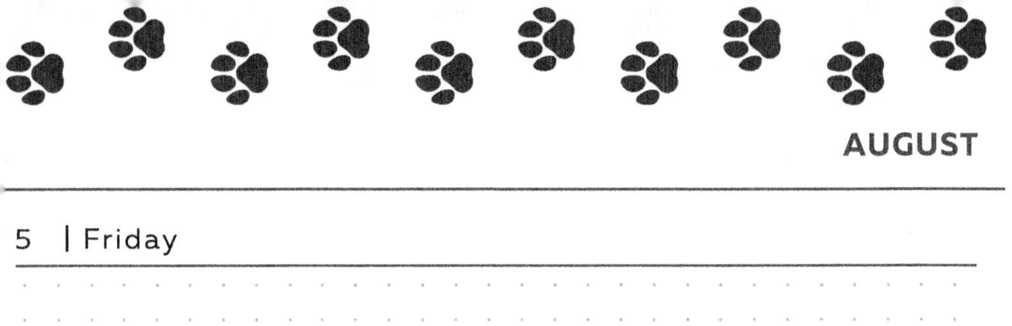

AUGUST

5 | Friday

6 | Saturday

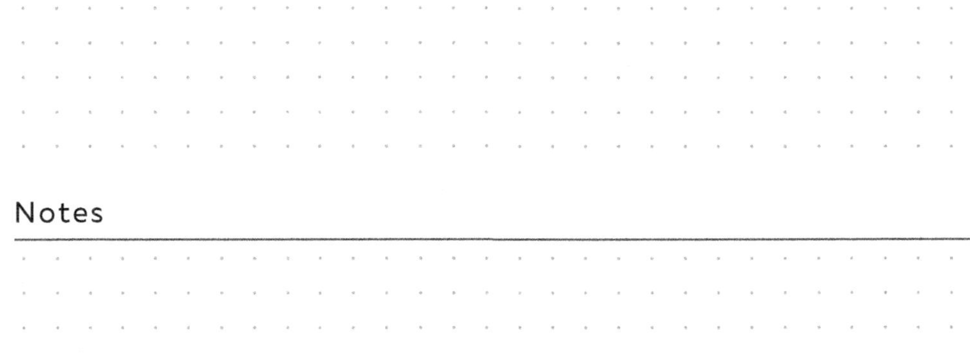

7 | Sunday

Notes

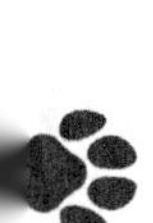
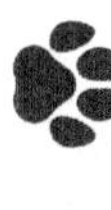
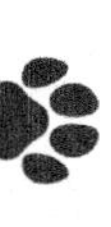
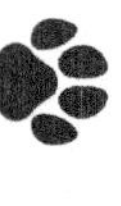
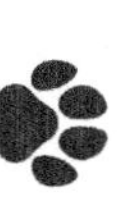

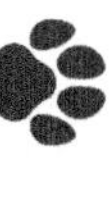
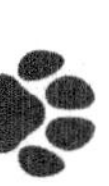
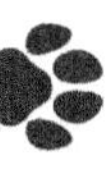
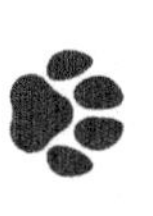
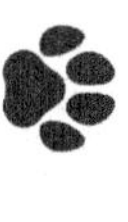

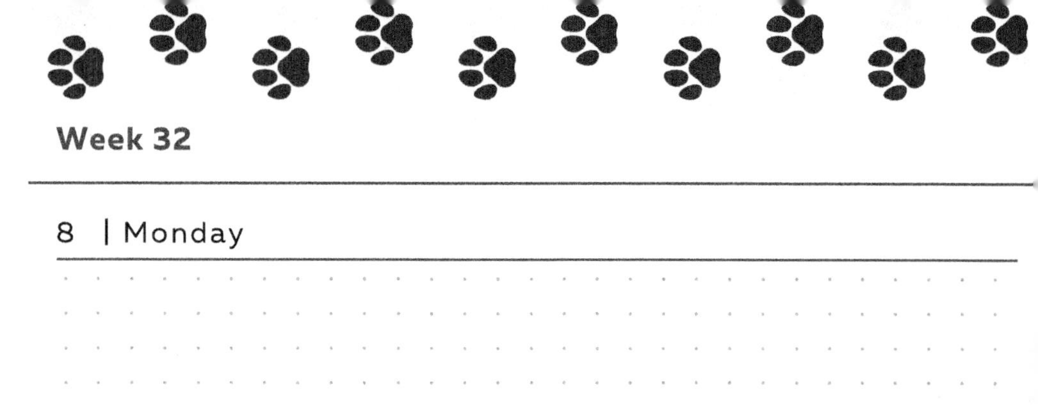

## Week 32

8 | Monday

9 | Tuesday

10 | Wednesday

11 | Thursday

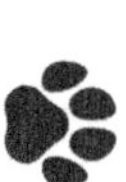
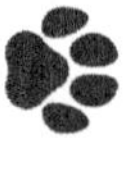
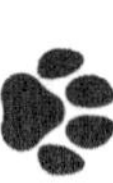

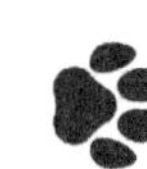
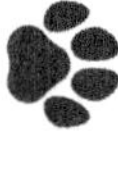
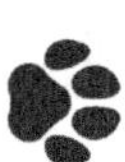
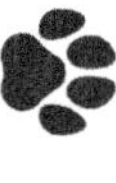
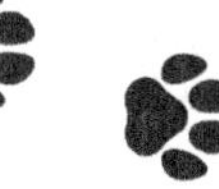
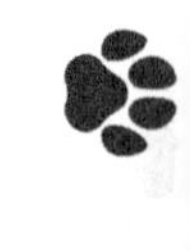

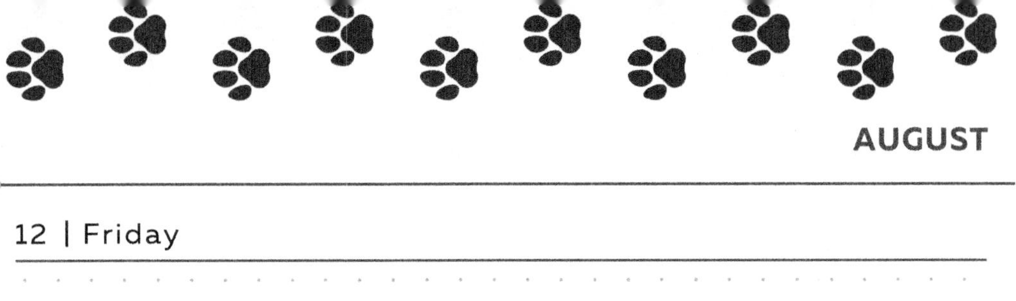

AUGUST

## 12 | Friday

## 13 | Saturday

## 14 | Sunday

## Notes

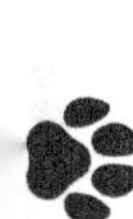
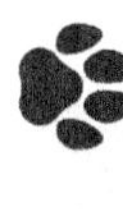
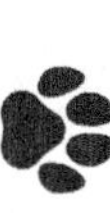

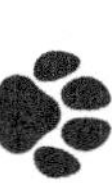
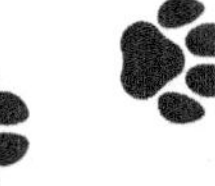
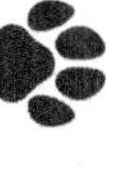
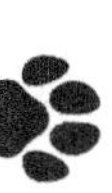

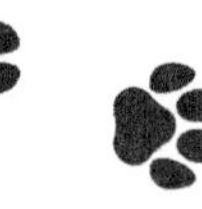
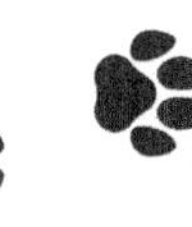

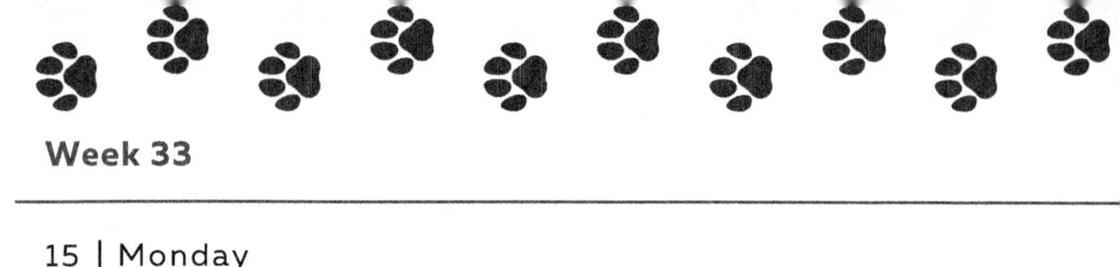

## Week 33

15 | Monday

16 | Tuesday

17 | Wednesday

18 | Thursday

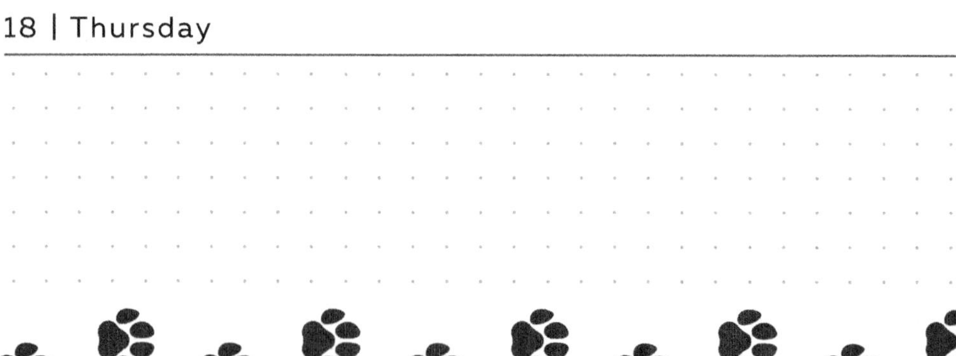
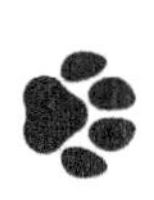
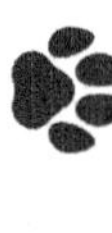
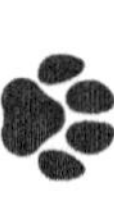
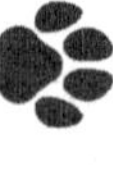
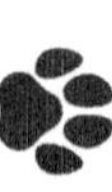
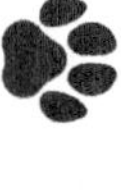
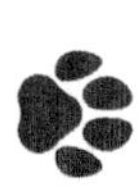
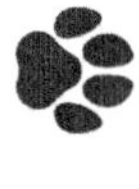
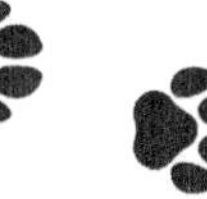
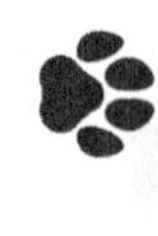

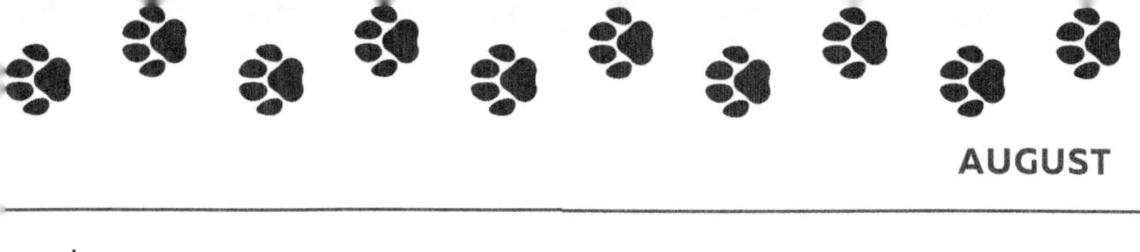



19 | Friday

20 | Saturday

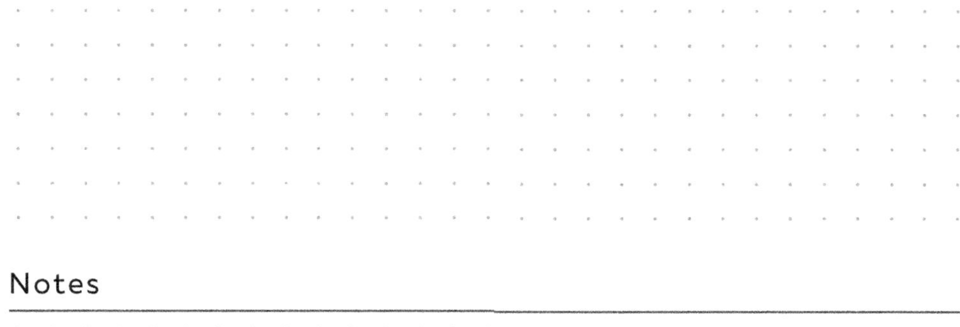

21 | Sunday

Notes

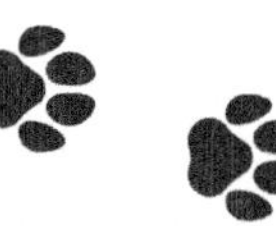
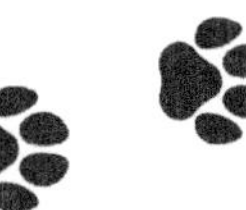
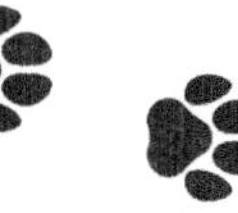
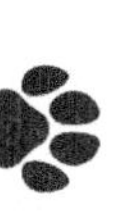
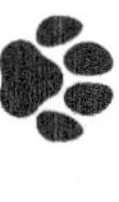
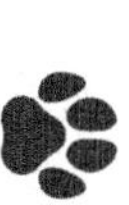
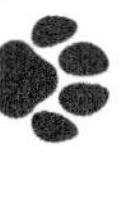

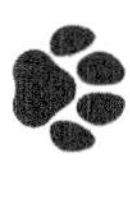

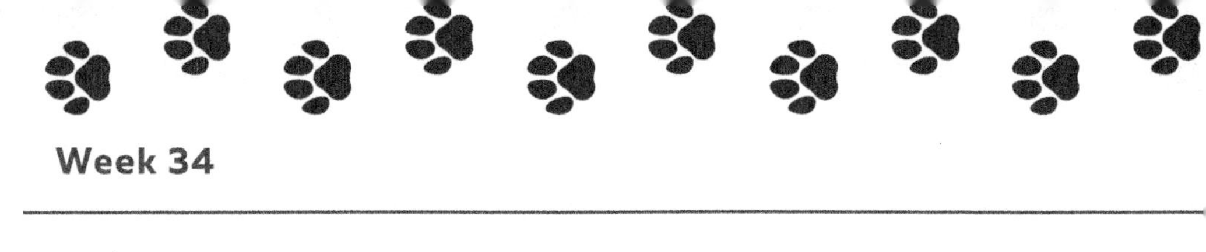

## Week 34

22 | Monday

23 | Tuesday

24 | Wednesday

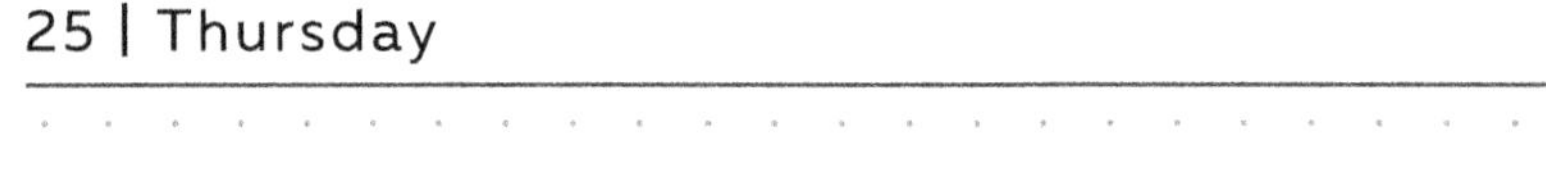

25 | Thursday

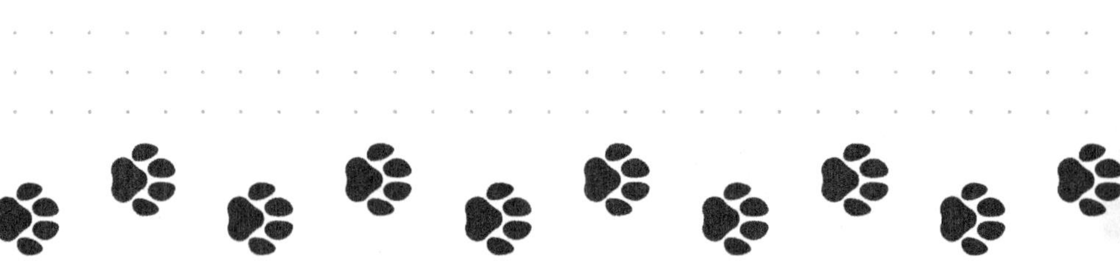

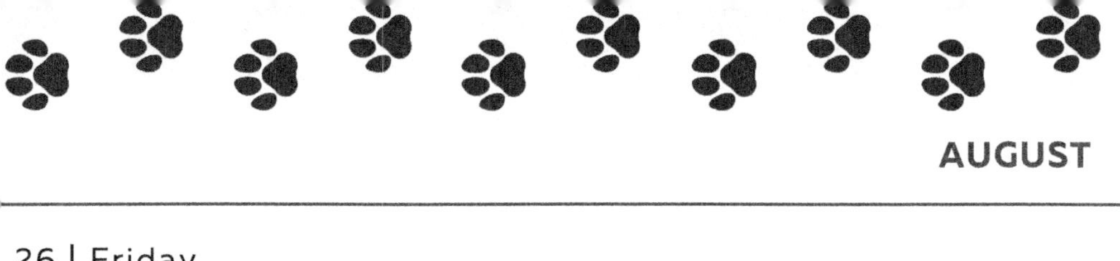



## 26 | Friday

## 27 | Saturday

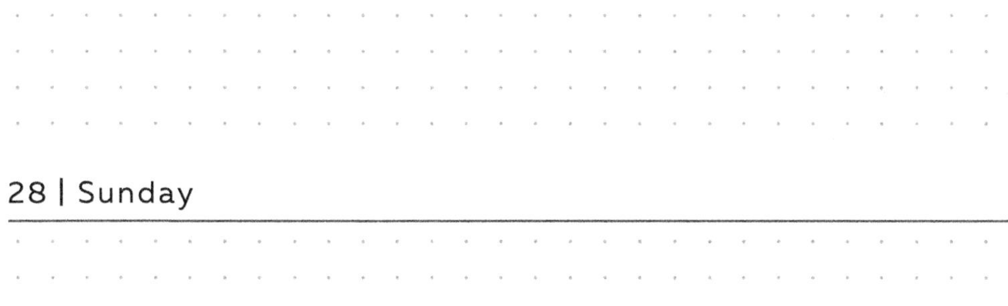

## 28 | Sunday

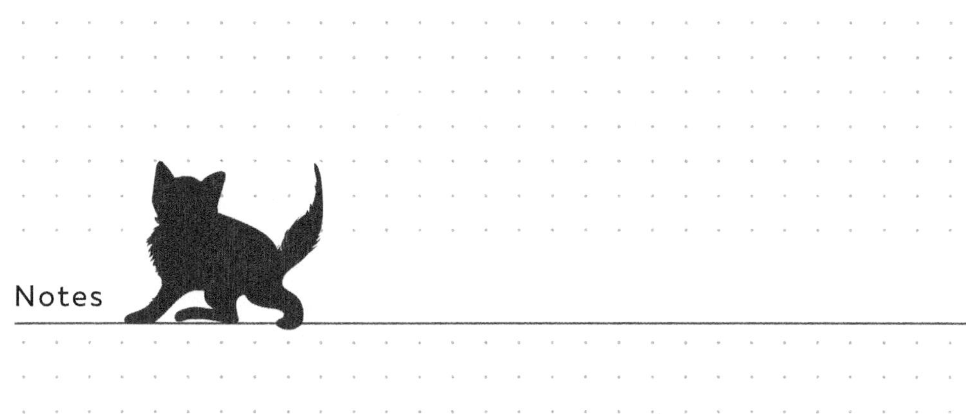

## Notes

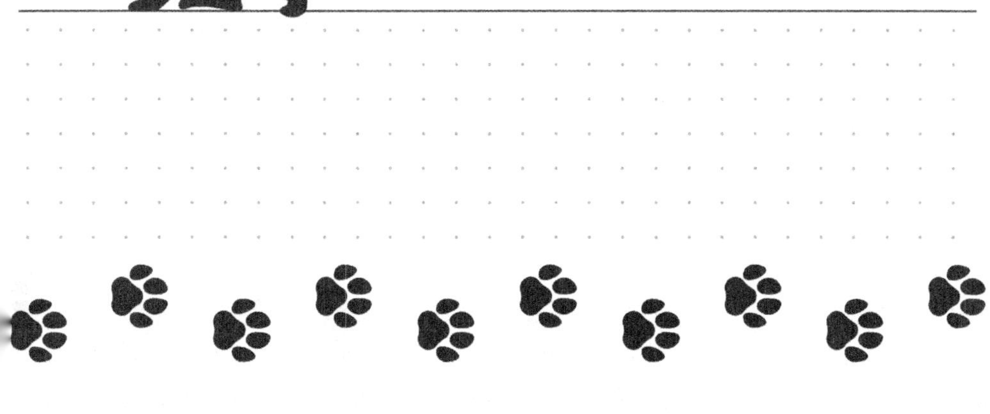

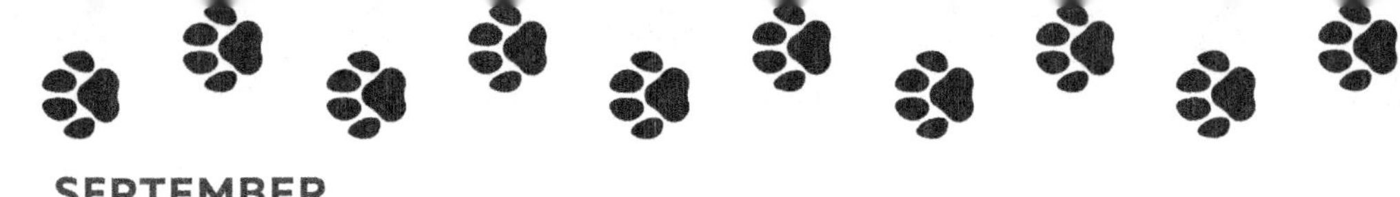

## SEPTEMBER

| Monday | Tuesday | Wednesday | Thursday |
| --- | --- | --- | --- |
| | | | 1 |
| 5 | 6 | 7 | 8 |
| 12 | 13 | 14 | 15 |
| 19 | 20 | 21 | 22 |
| 26 | 27 | 28 | 29 |

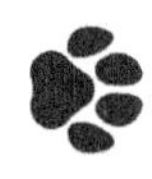

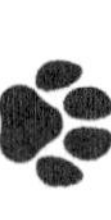

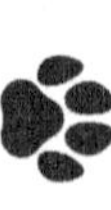
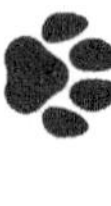
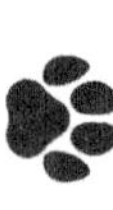
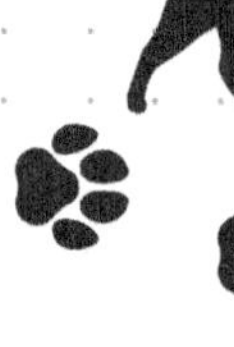
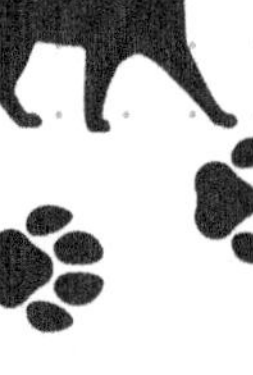

2022

| Friday | Saturday | Sunday |
|---|---|---|
| 2 | 3 | 4 |
| 9 | 10 | 11 |
| 16 | 17 | 18 |
| 23 | 24 | 25 |
| 30 | | |

Goals

To Do

Reminder

Notes

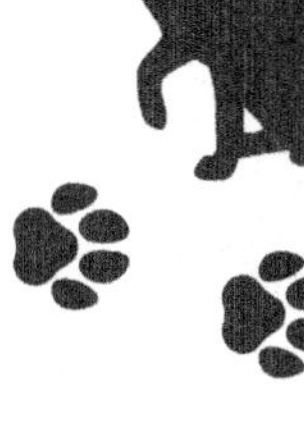

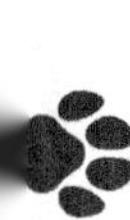
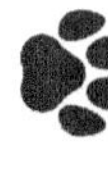
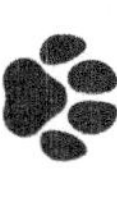
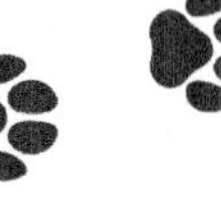
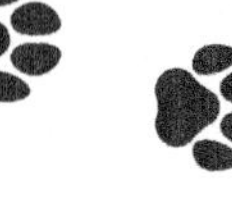
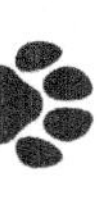

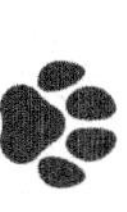
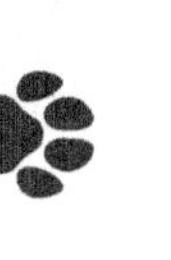

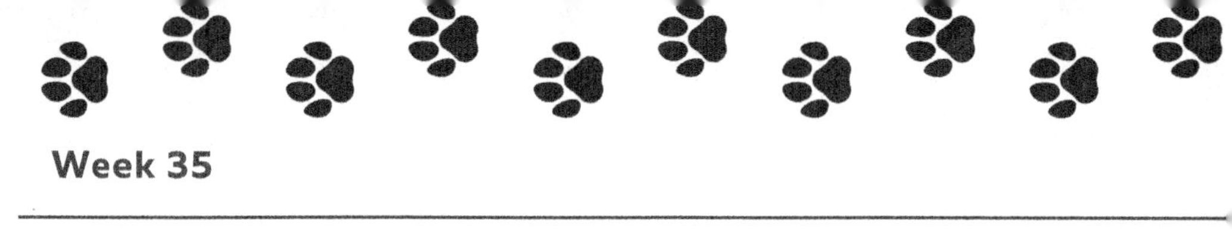

## Week 35

### 29 | Monday

### 30 | Tuesday

### 31 | Wednesday

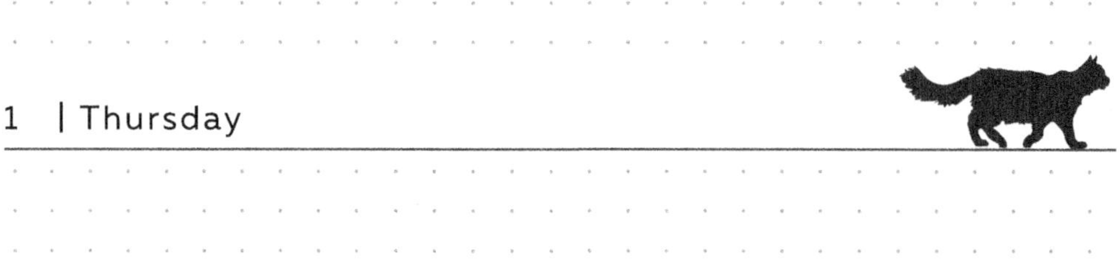

### 1 | Thursday

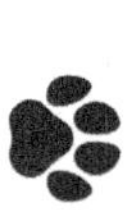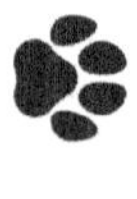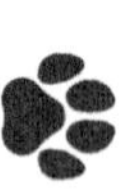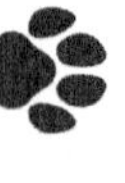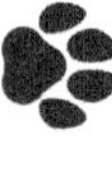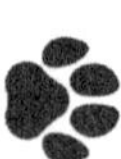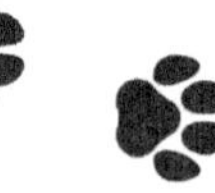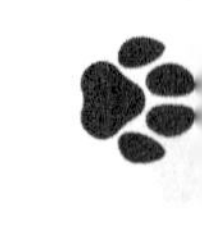

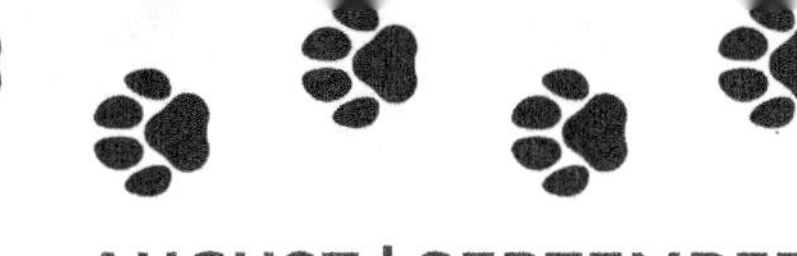



## 2 | Friday

## 3 | Saturday

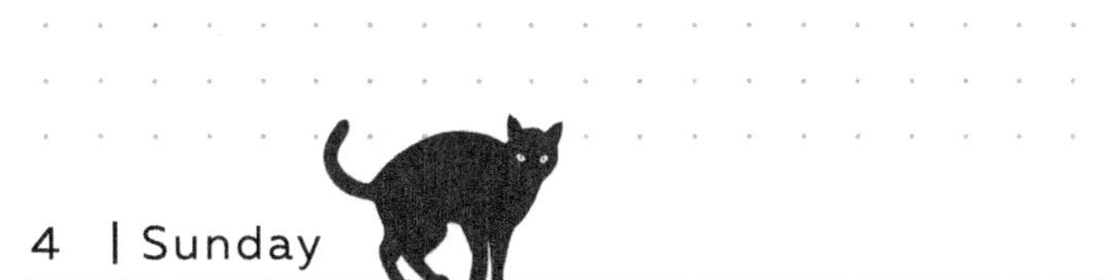

## 4 | Sunday

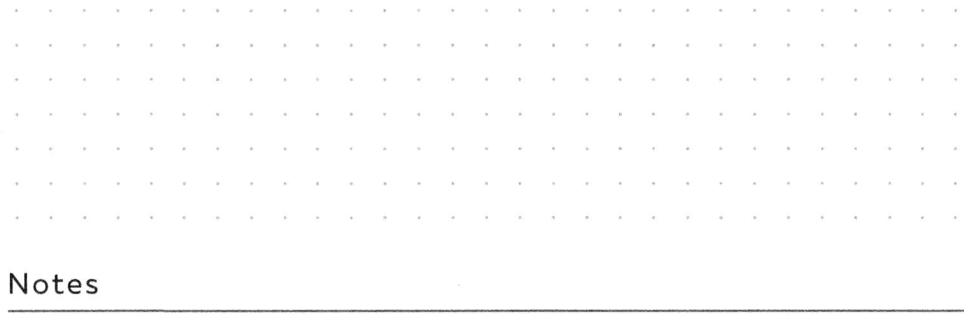

## Notes

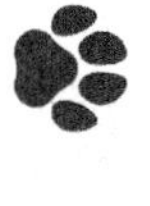
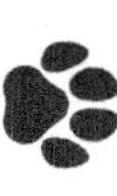
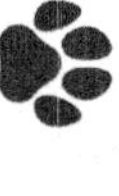
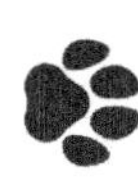

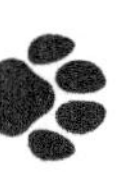

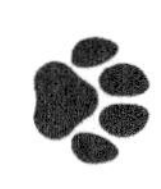
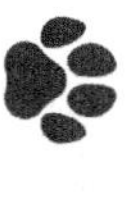

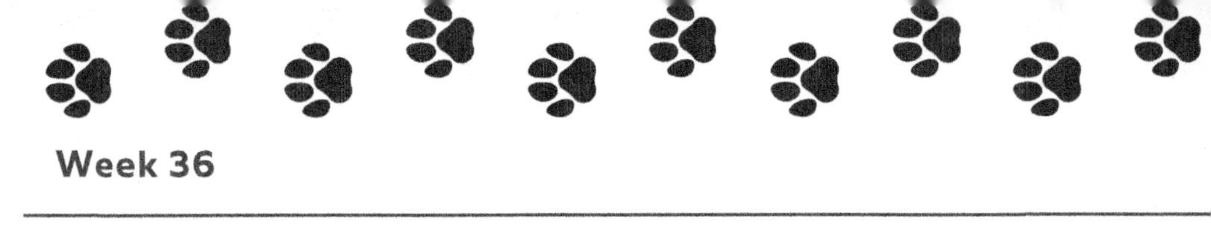

## Week 36

### 5 | Monday

### 6 | Tuesday

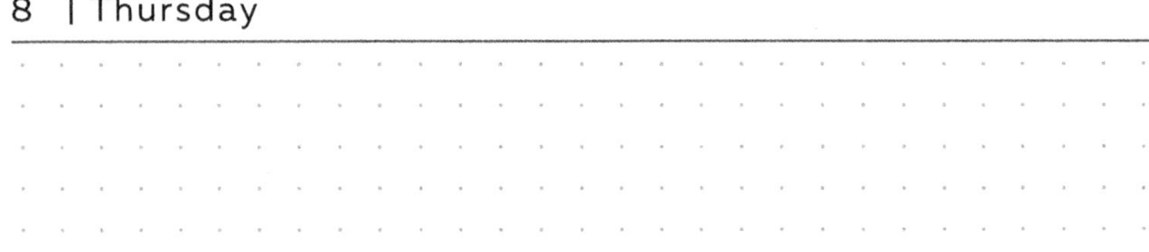

### 7 | Wednesday

### 8 | Thursday

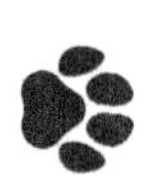
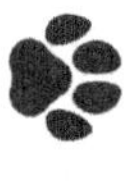
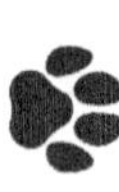
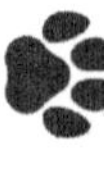
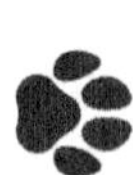

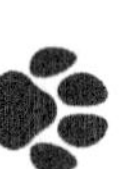
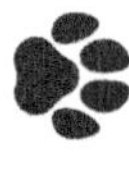
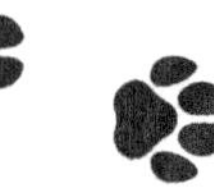
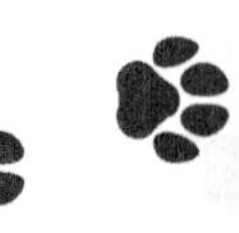

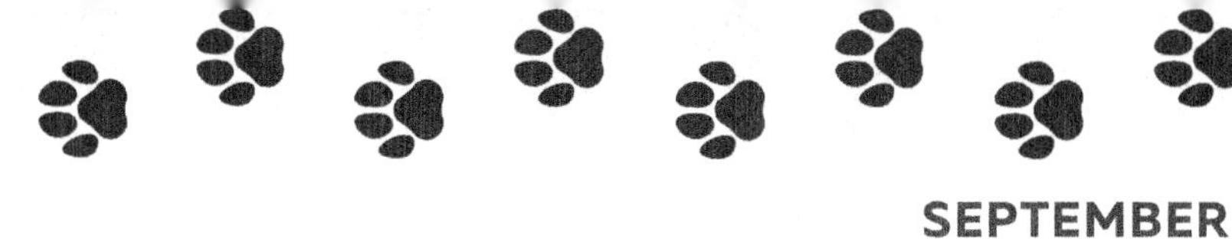



9 | Friday

10 | Saturday

11 | Sunday

Notes

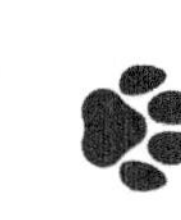
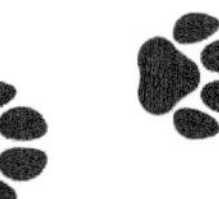
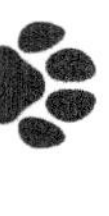
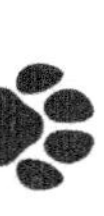
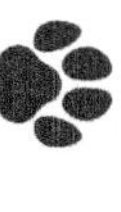
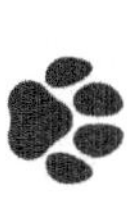
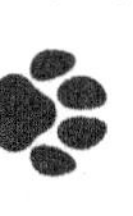
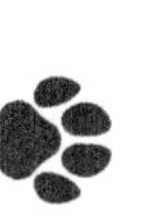
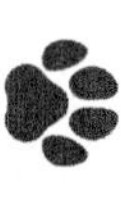

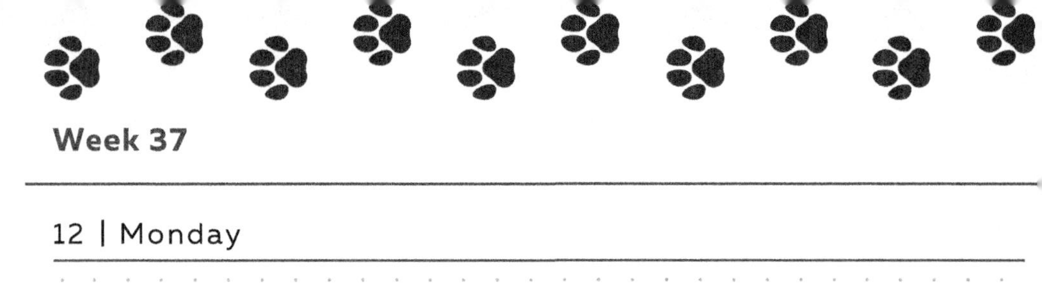

## Week 37

### 12 | Monday

### 13 | Tuesday

### 14 | Wednesday

### 15 | Thursday

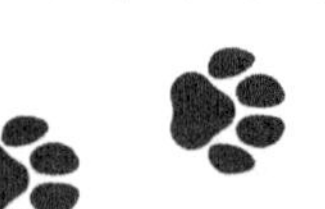
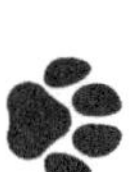
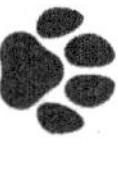

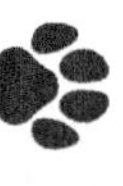
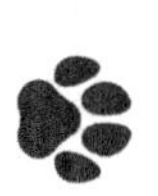
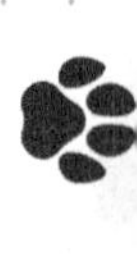

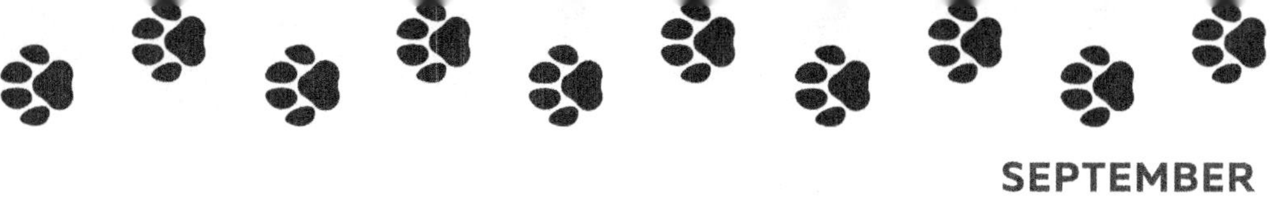

SEPTEMBER

16 | Friday

17 | Saturday

18 | Sunday

Notes

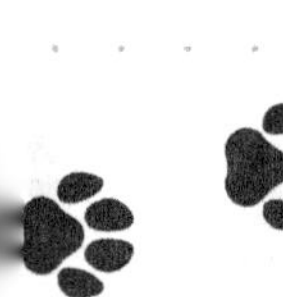
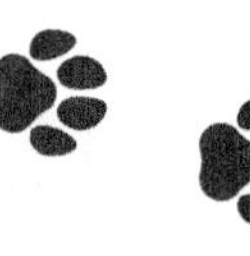
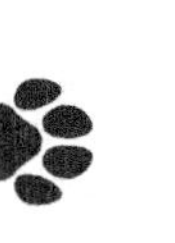
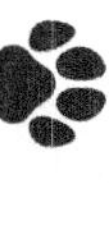
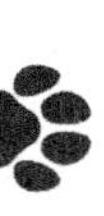

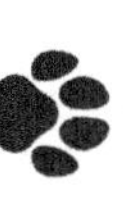
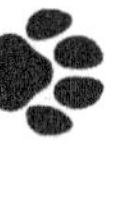
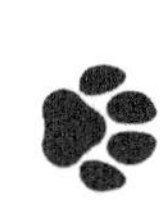
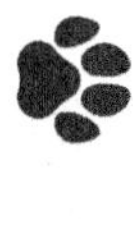

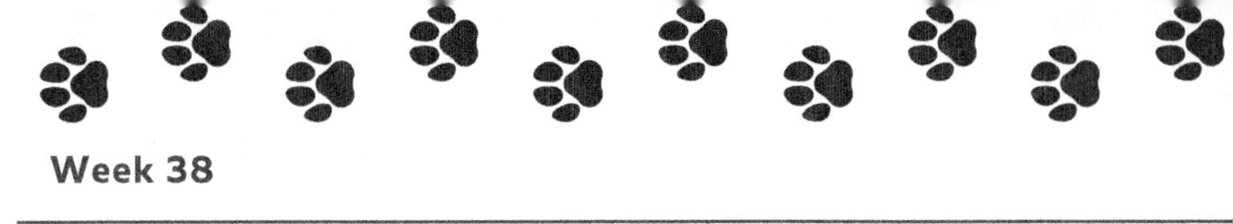

## Week 38

19 | Monday

20 | Tuesday

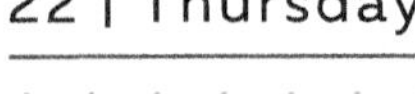

21 | Wednesday

22 | Thursday

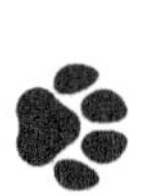
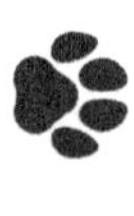
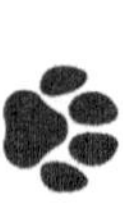

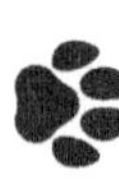
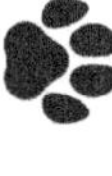
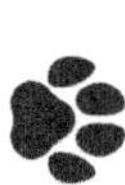
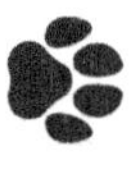
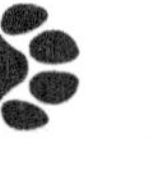
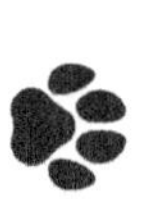
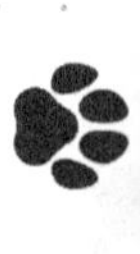

## SEPTEMBER

### 23 | Friday

### 24 | Saturday

### 25 | Sunday

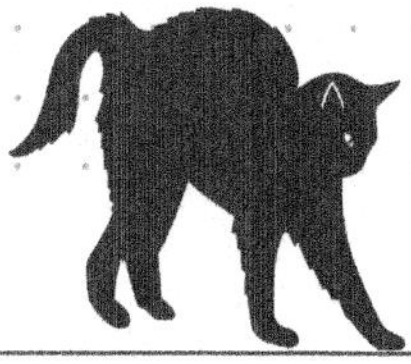

### Notes

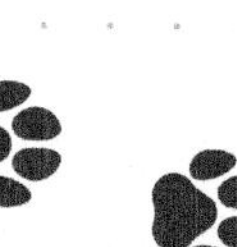

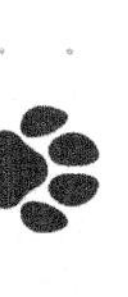

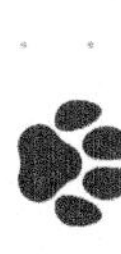

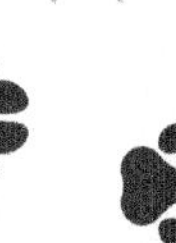

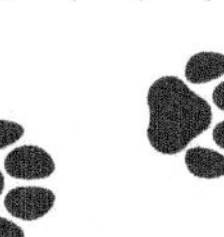

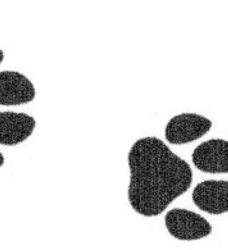

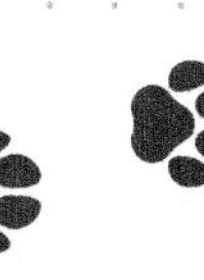

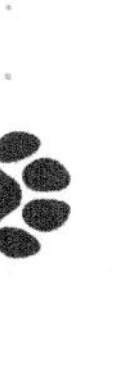

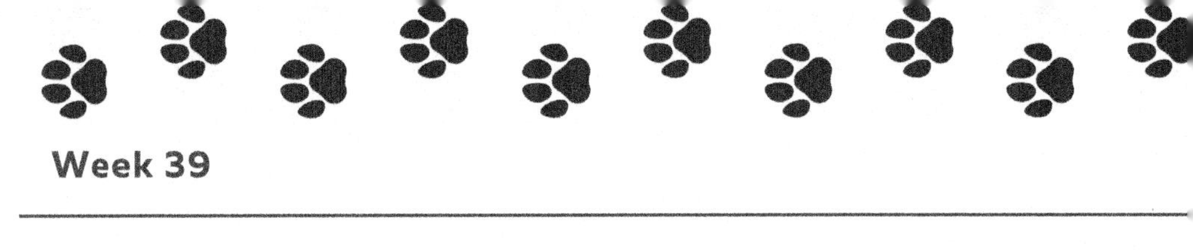

## Week 39

26 | Monday

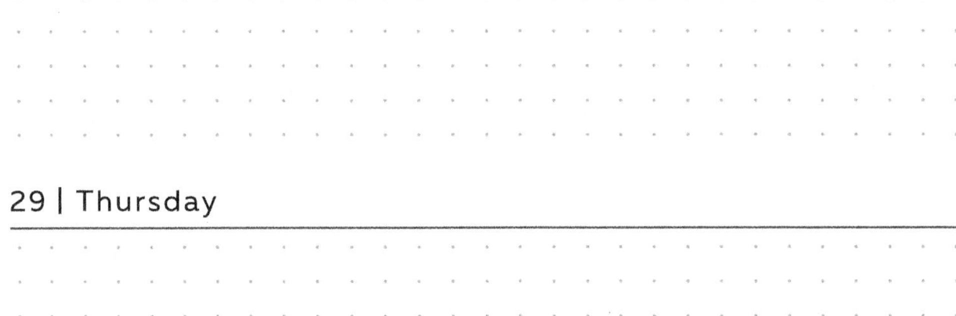

27 | Tuesday

28 | Wednesday

29 | Thursday

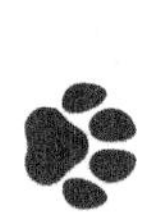 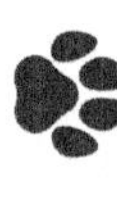 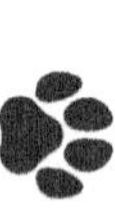 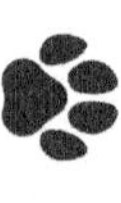 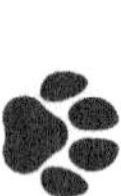 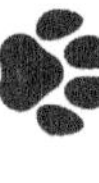 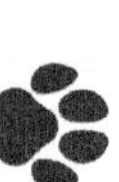 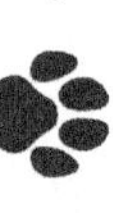 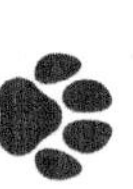 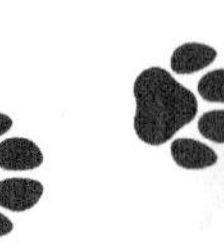

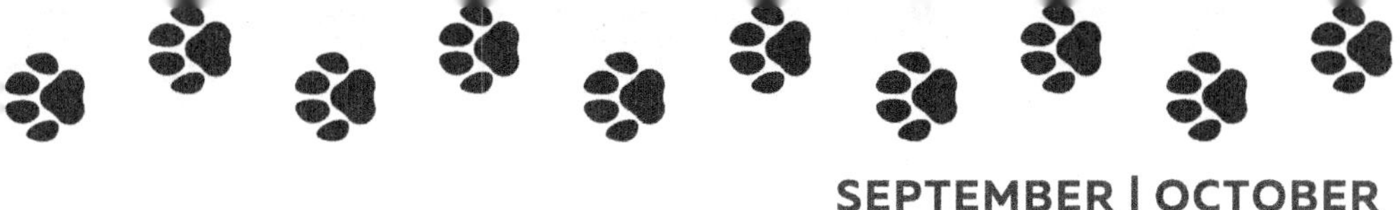



30 | Friday

1 | Saturday

2 | Sunday

Notes

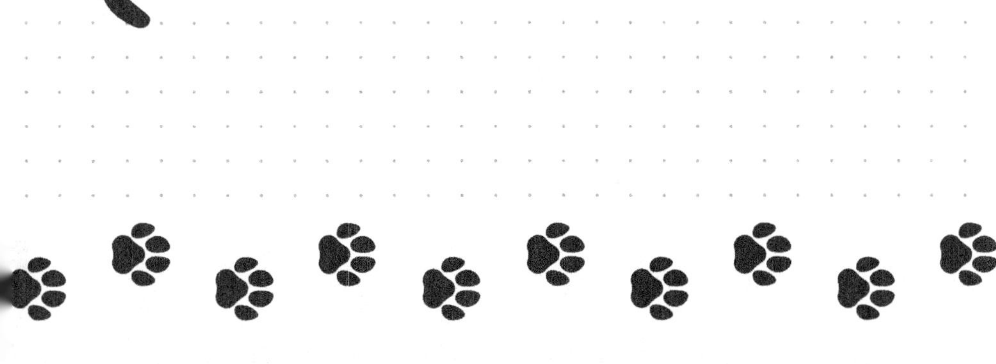

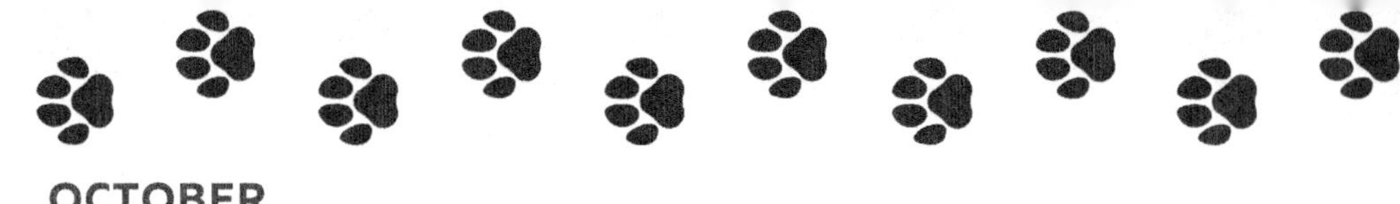

## OCTOBER

| Monday | Tuesday | Wednesday | Thursday |
| --- | --- | --- | --- |
| | | | |
| 3 | 4 | 5 | 6 |
| 10 | 11 | 12 | 13 |
| 17 | 18 | 19 | 20 |
| 24 | 25 | 26 | 27 |
| 31 Halloween | | | |

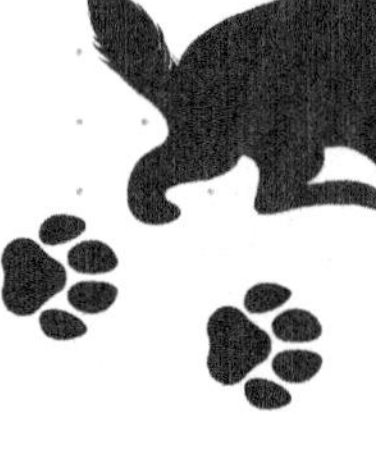

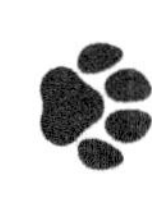
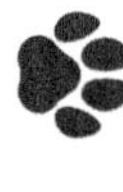
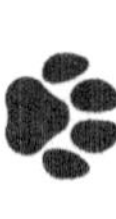
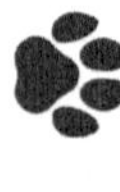
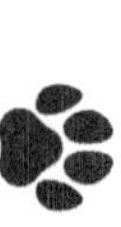
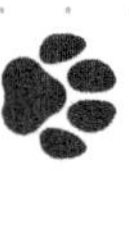
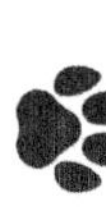

2022

| Friday | Saturday | Sunday |
| --- | --- | --- |
| | 1 | 2 |
| 7 | 8 | 9 |
| 14 | 15 | 16 |
| 21 | 22 | 23 |
| 28 | 29 | 30 |

Goals

To Do

Reminder

Notes

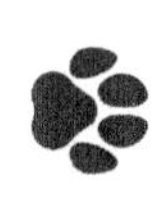
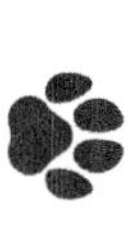
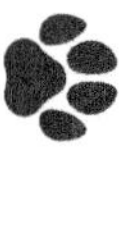
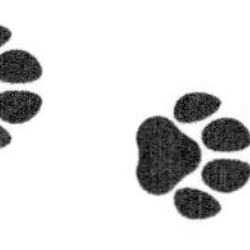

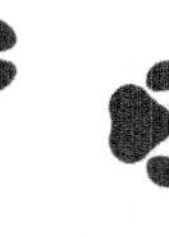

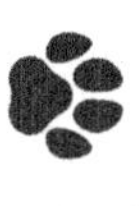
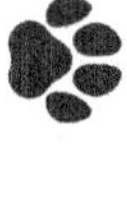

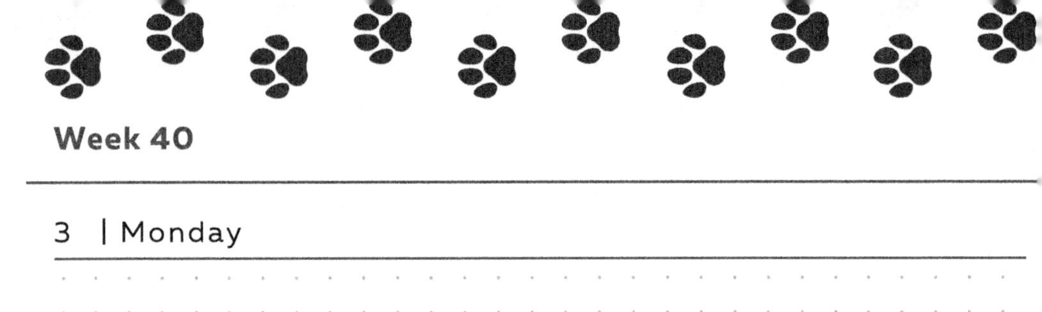

## Week 40

### 3 | Monday

### 4 | Tuesday

### 5 | Wednesday

### 6 | Thursday

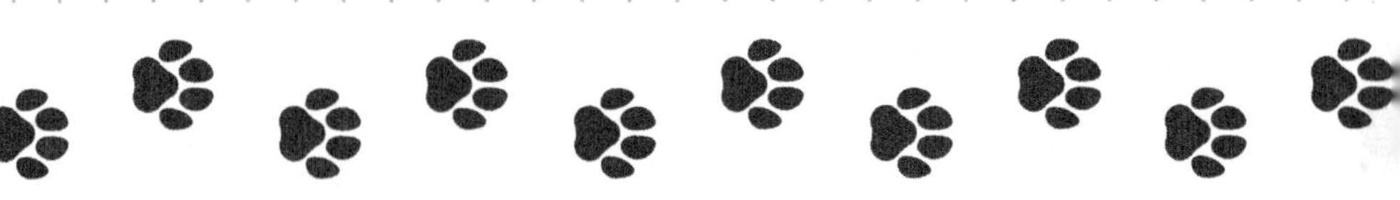

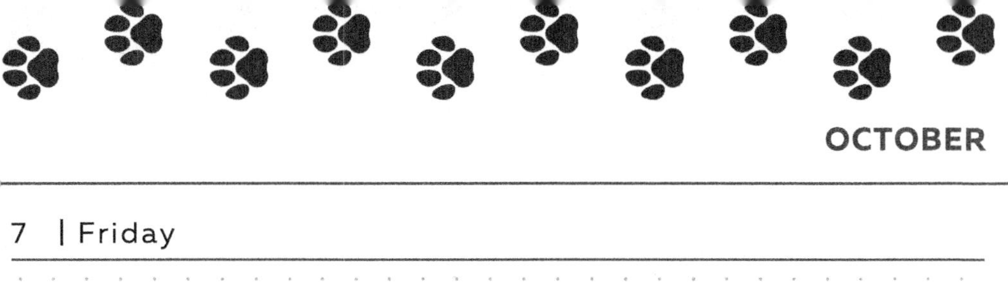



7 | Friday

8 | Saturday

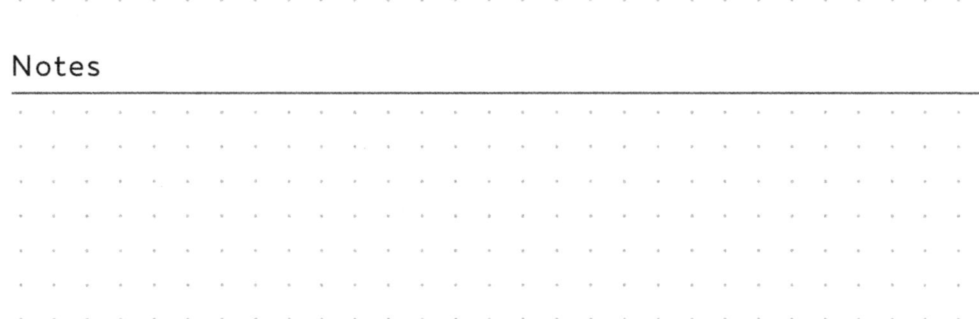

9 | Sunday

Notes

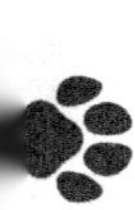
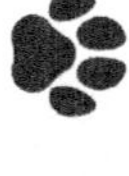
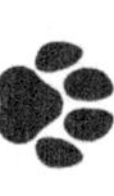
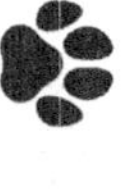
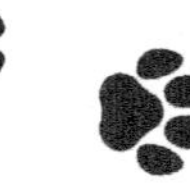
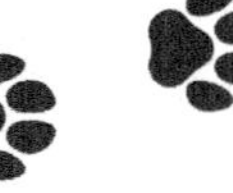

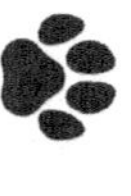
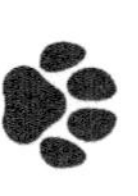
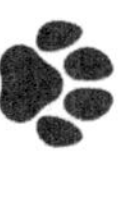

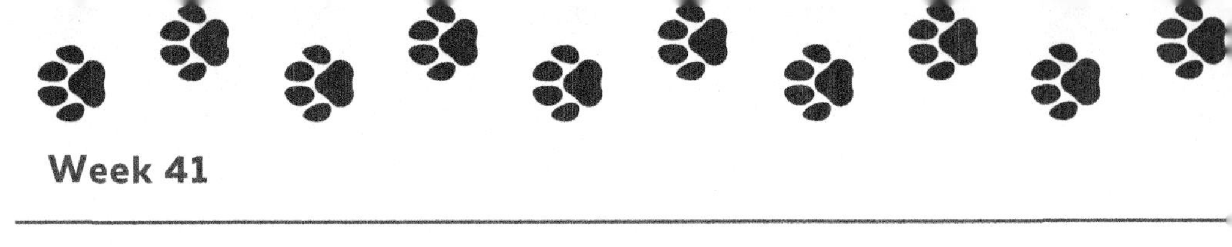

## Week 41

### 10 | Monday

### 11 | Tuesday

### 12 | Wednesday

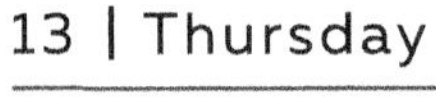

### 13 | Thursday

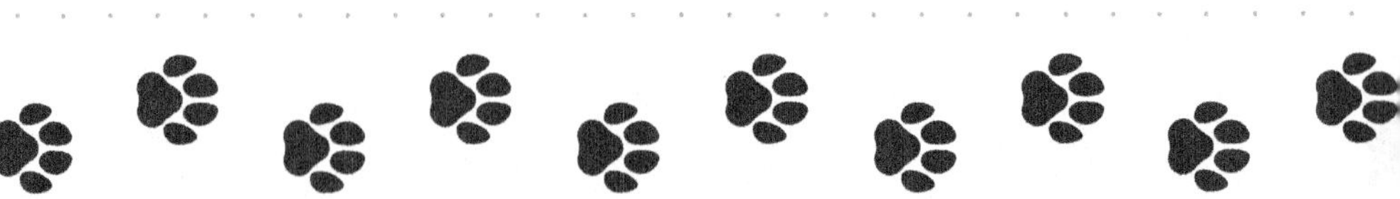

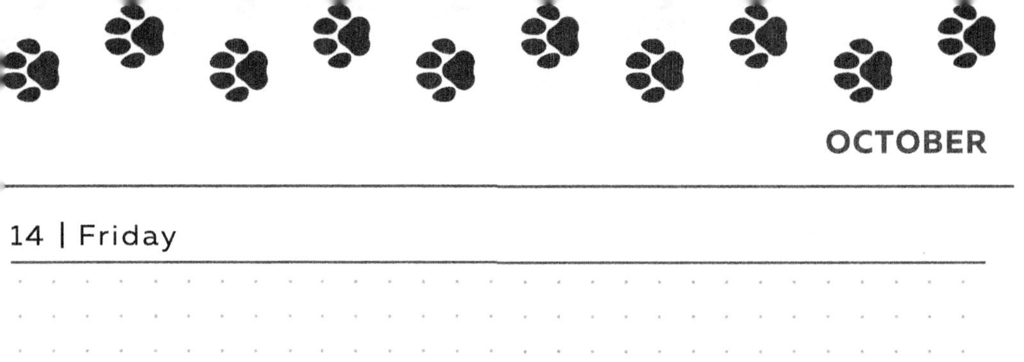



14 | Friday

15 | Saturday

16 | Sunday

Notes

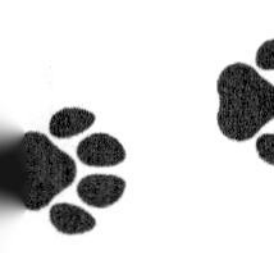
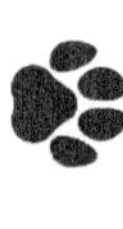
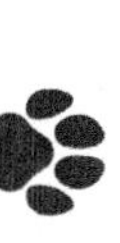
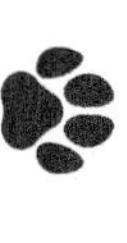
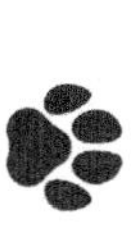
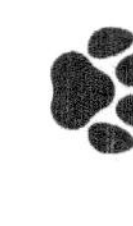
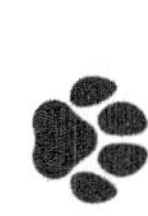
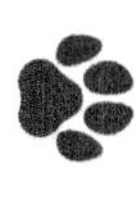
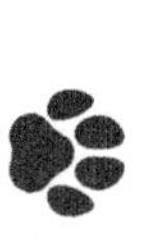
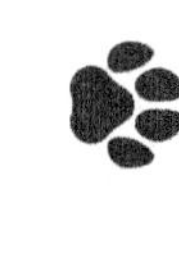

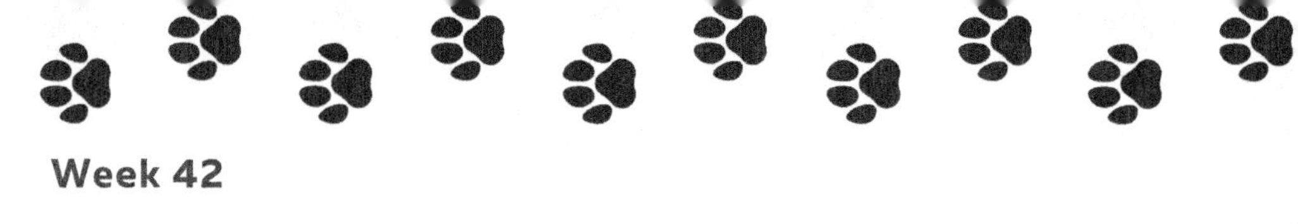

## Week 42

17 | Monday

18 | Tuesday

19 | Wednesday

20 | Thursday

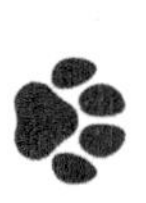
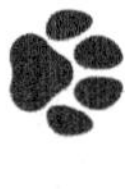
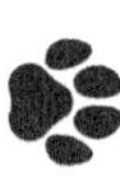
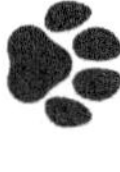
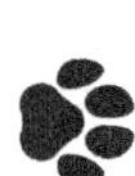
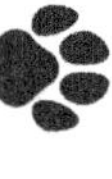
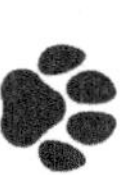
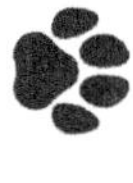
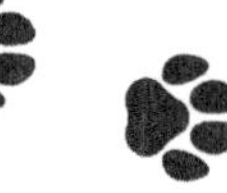
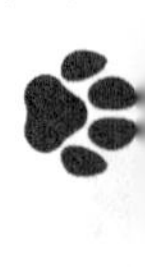

21 | Friday

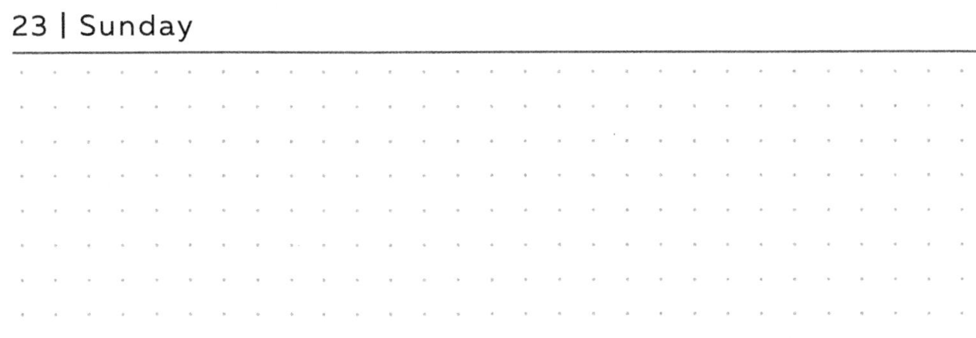

22 | Saturday

23 | Sunday

Notes

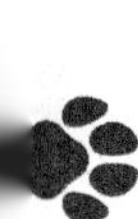
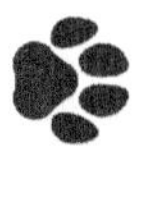
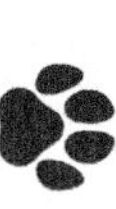

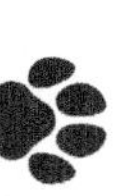
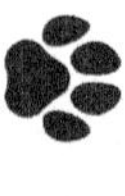
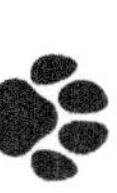
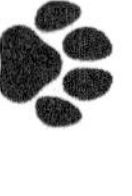
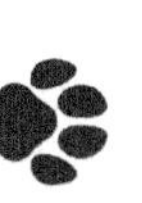
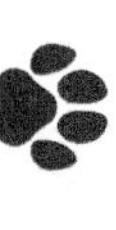

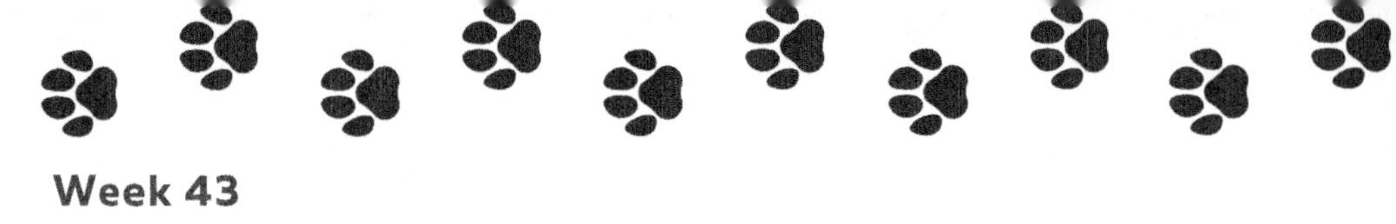

## Week 43

### 24 | Monday

### 25 | Tuesday

### 26 | Wednesday

### 27 | Thursday

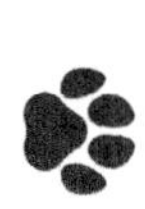
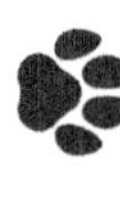
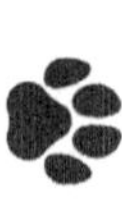
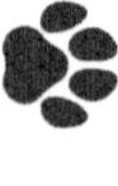

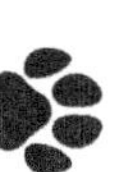
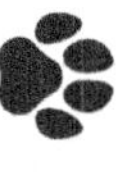
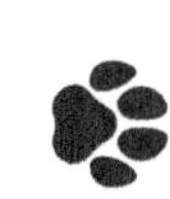
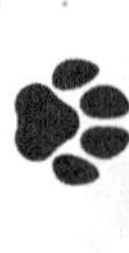

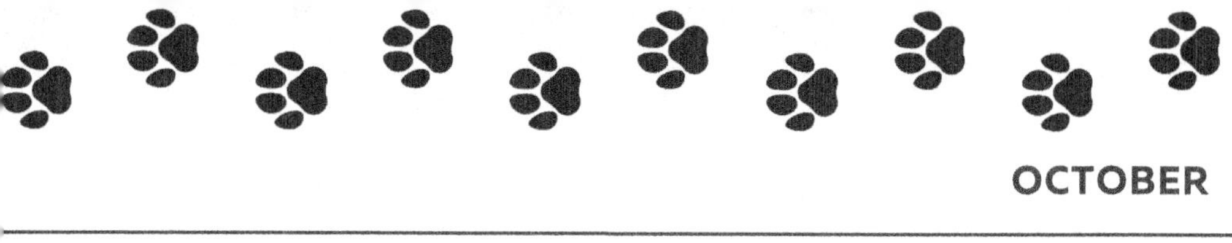

OCTOBER

28 | Friday

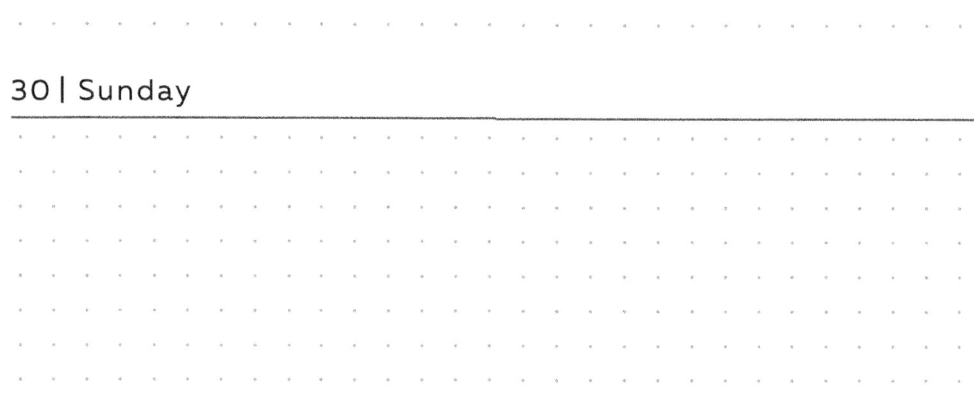

29 | Saturday

30 | Sunday

Notes

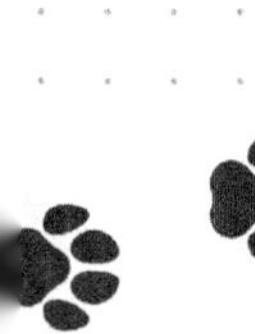
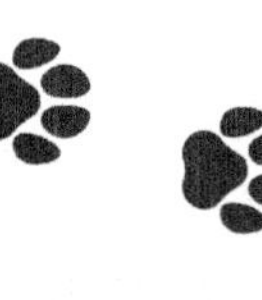
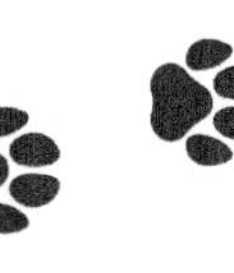
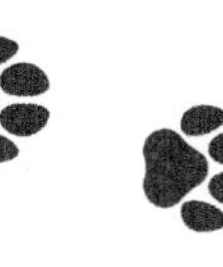

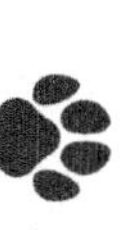
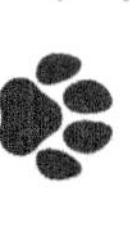

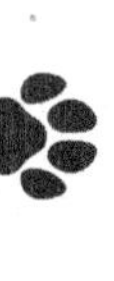

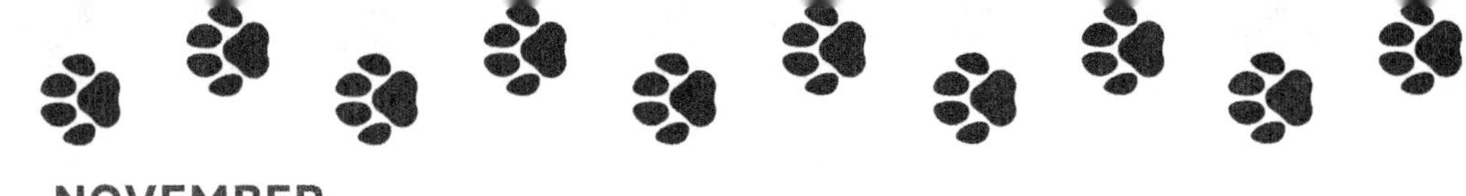

## NOVEMBER

| Monday | Tuesday | Wednesday | Thursday |
| --- | --- | --- | --- |
| | 1 | 2 | 3 |
| 7 | 8 | 9 | 10 |
| 14 | 15 | 16 | 17 |
| 21 | 22 | 23 | 24 |
| 28 | 29 | 30 | |

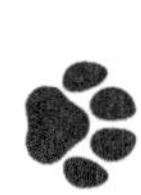 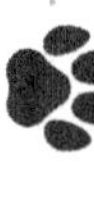 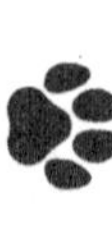 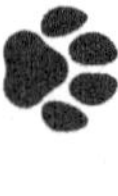   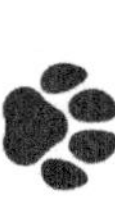 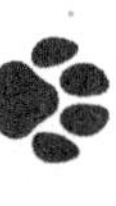 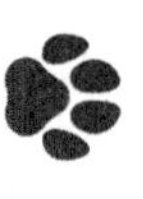 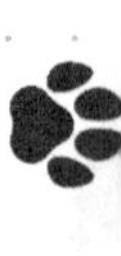

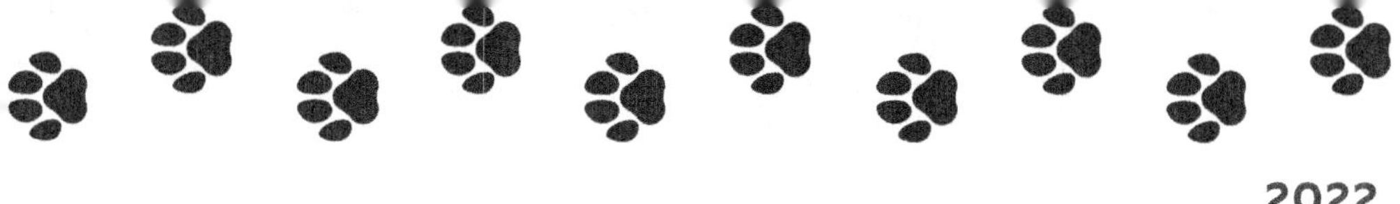

2022

| Friday | Saturday | Sunday |
| --- | --- | --- |
| 4 | 5 Guy Fawkes Day | 6 |
| 11 | 12 | 13 Remembrance Sunday |
| 18 | 19 | 20 |
| 25 | 26 | 27 |

## Goals

## To Do

## Reminder

## Notes

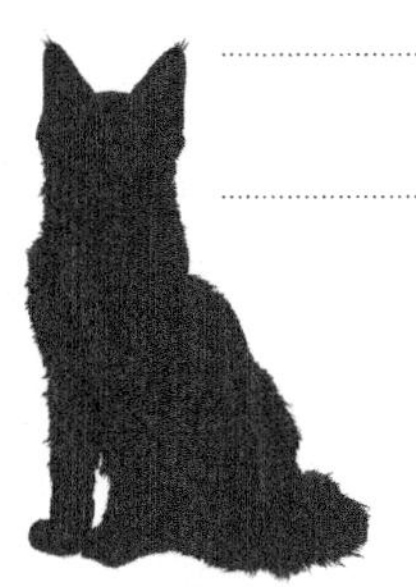

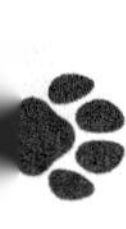 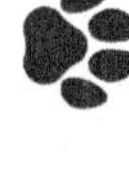 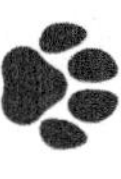 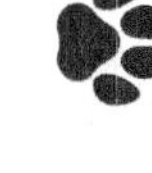  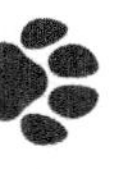  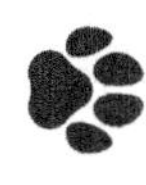 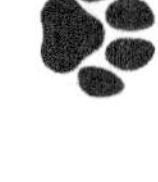  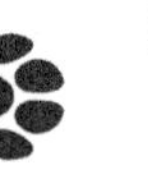 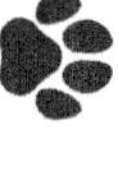

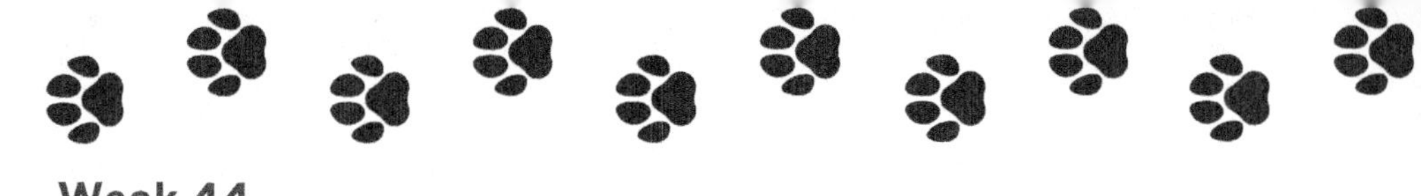

## Week 44

31 | Monday Halloween

1 | Tuesday

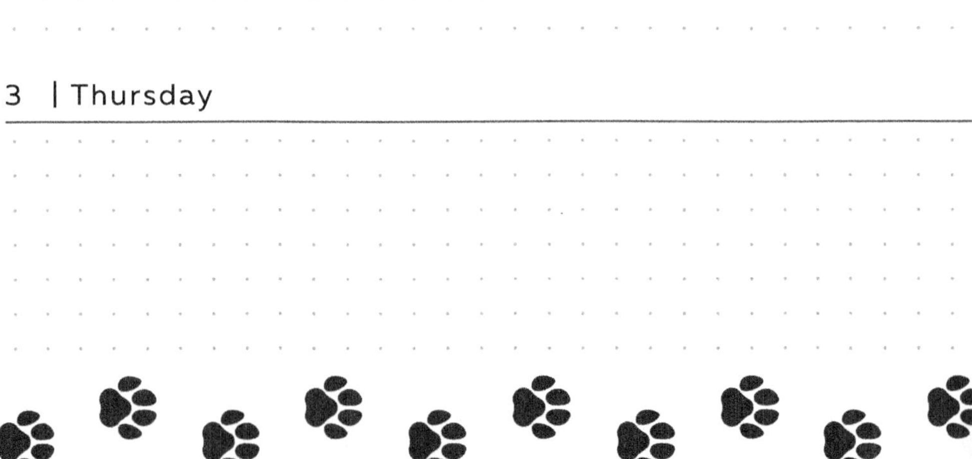

2 | Wednesday

3 | Thursday

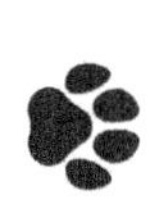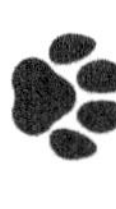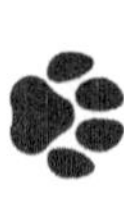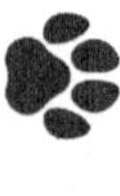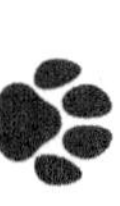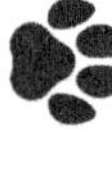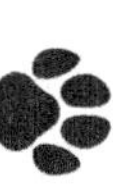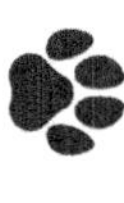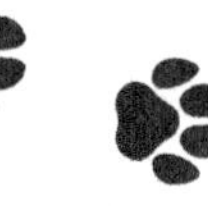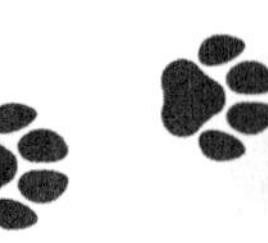

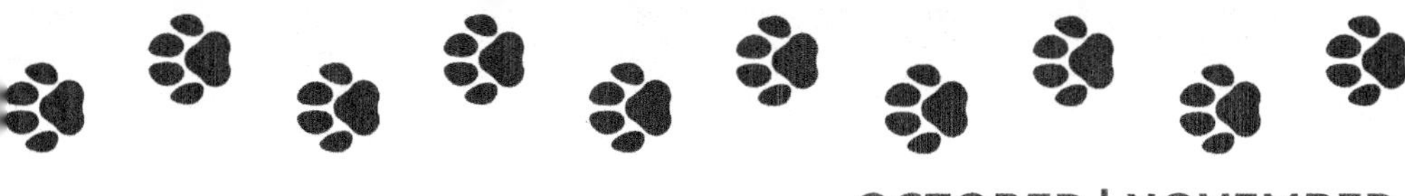



4 | Friday

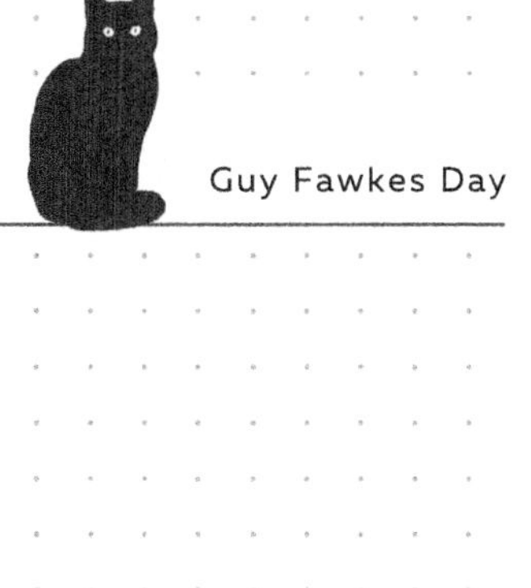

5 | Saturday

Guy Fawkes Day

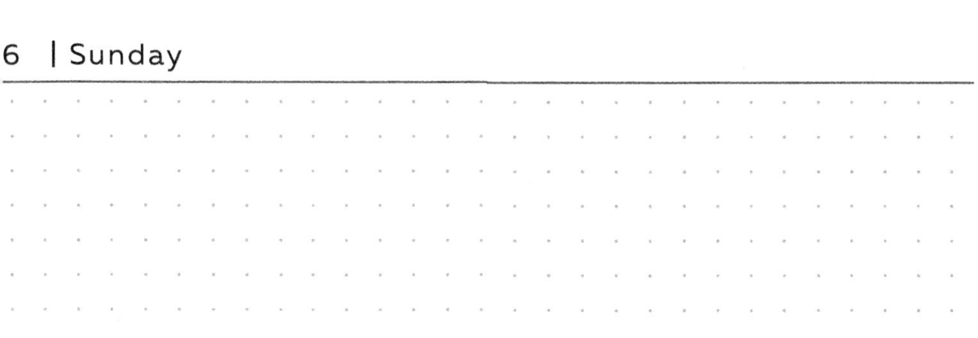

6 | Sunday

Notes

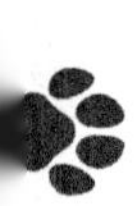 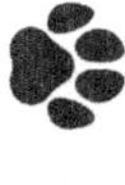 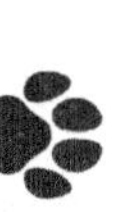 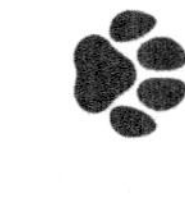 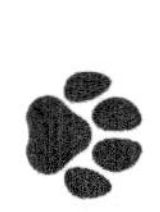 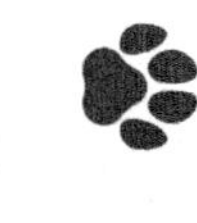 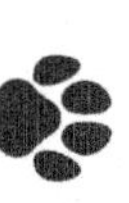 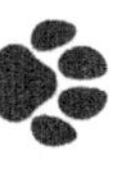 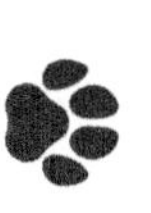 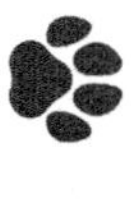

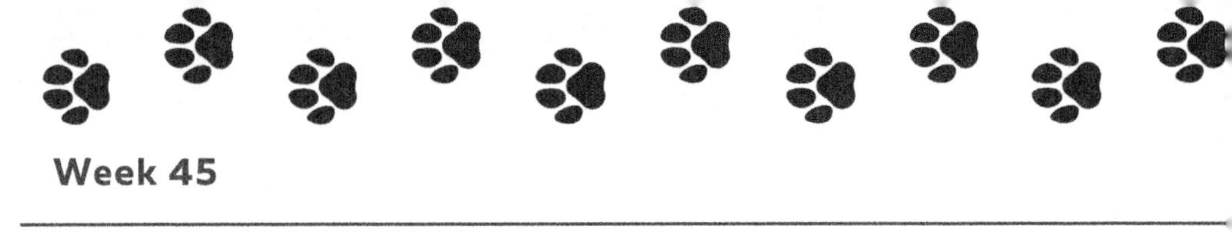

## Week 45

7 | Monday

8 | Tuesday

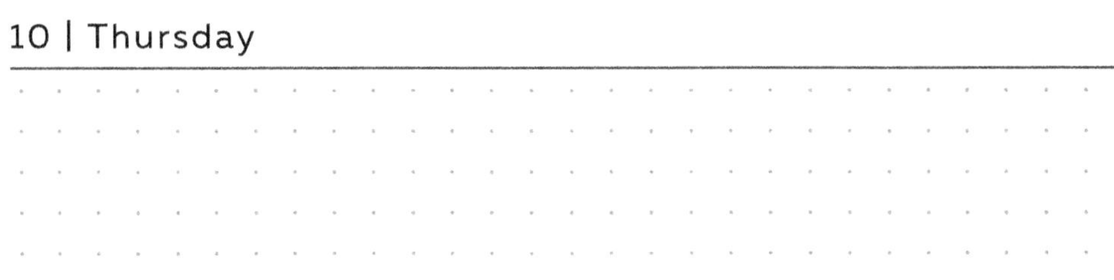

9 | Wednesday

10 | Thursday

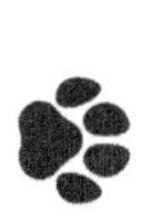
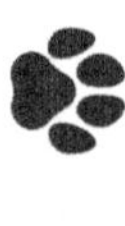
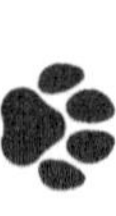
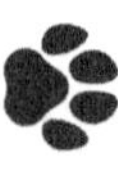

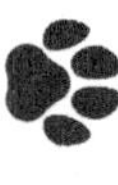

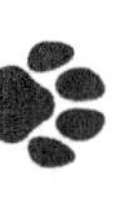
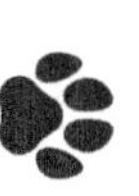
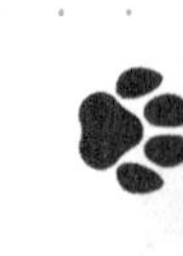

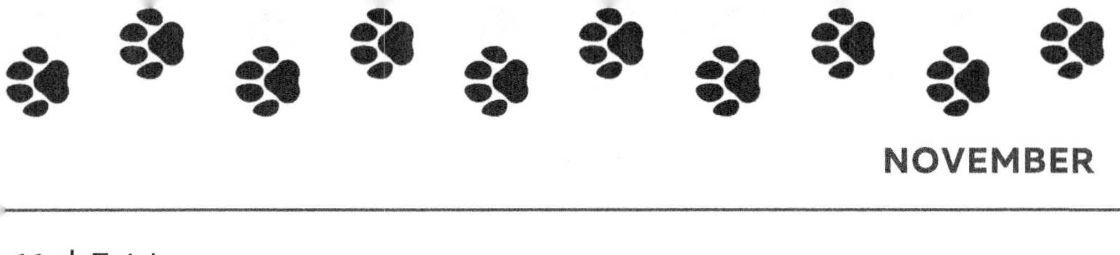



11 | Friday

12 | Saturday

13 | Sunday

Remembrance Sunday

Notes

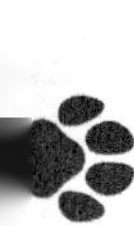
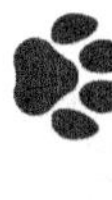
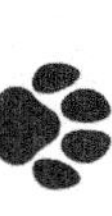
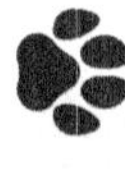
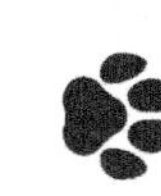
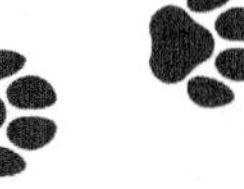
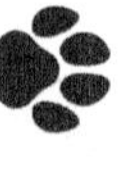
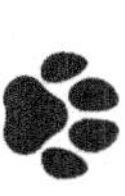
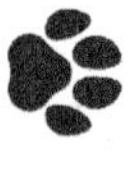
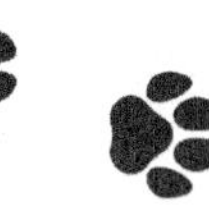
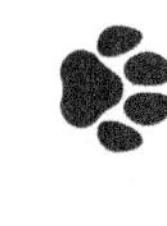

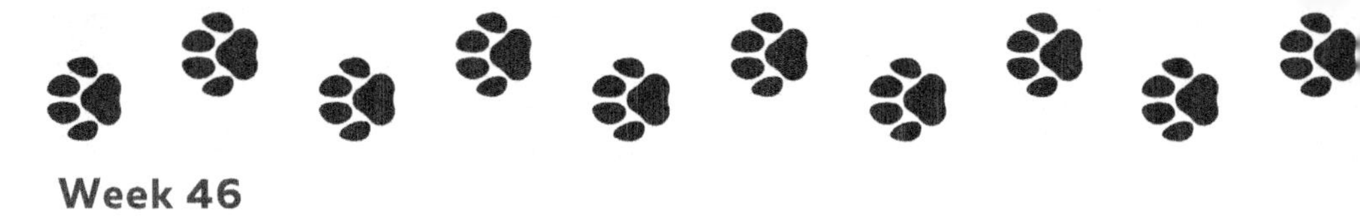

## Week 46

### 14 | Monday

### 15 | Tuesday

### 16 | Wednesday

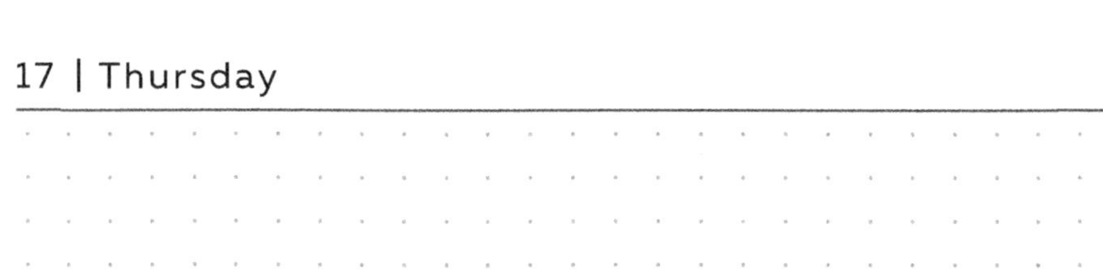

### 17 | Thursday

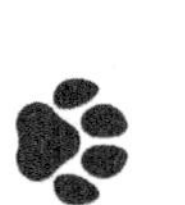  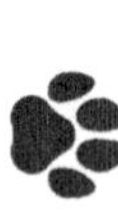 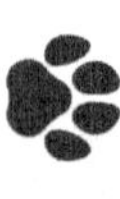 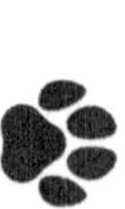 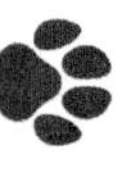 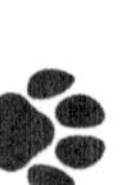 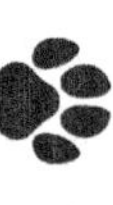  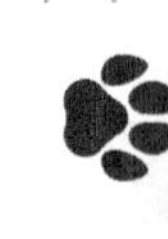

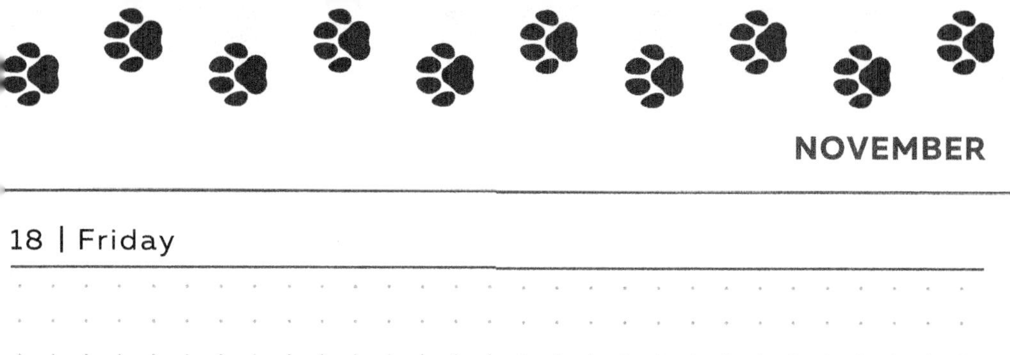

NOVEMBER

18 | Friday

19 | Saturday

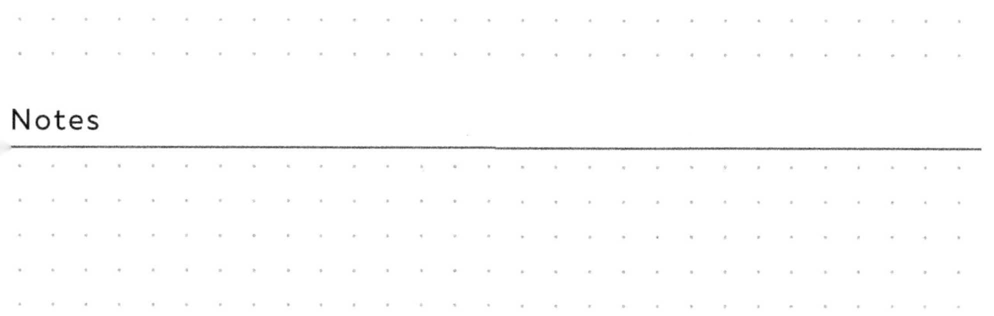

20 | Sunday

Notes

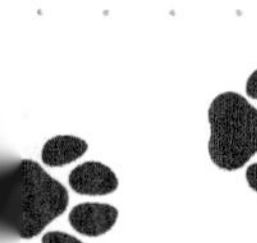
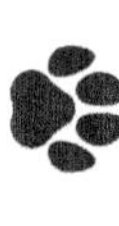
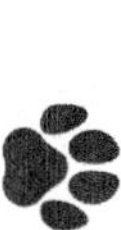
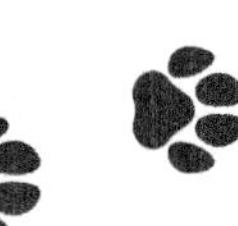
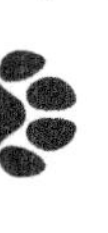

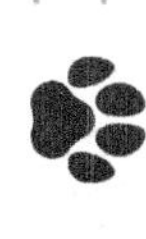

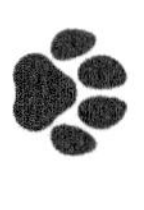
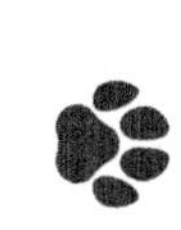
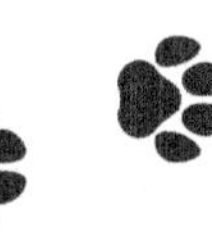

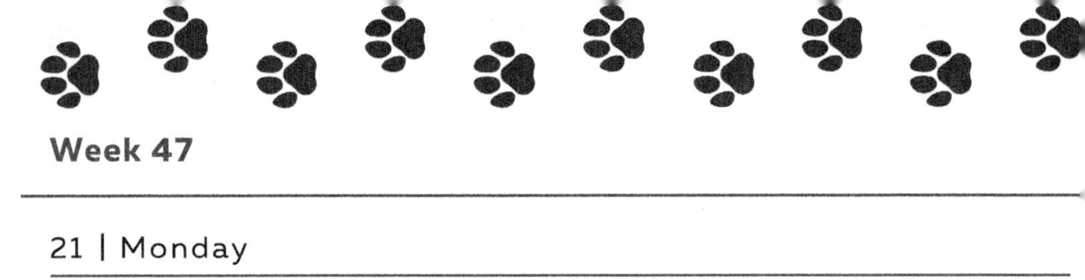

## Week 47

21 | Monday

22 | Tuesday

23 | Wednesday

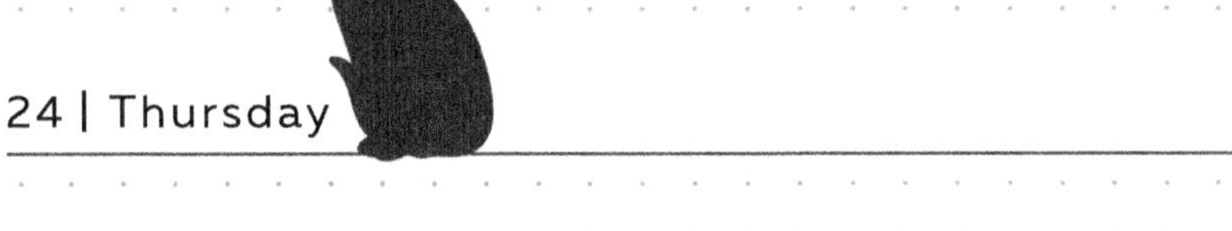

24 | Thursday

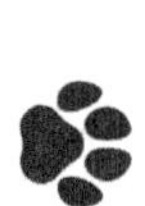
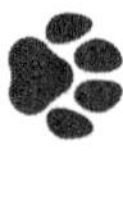
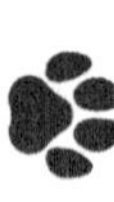
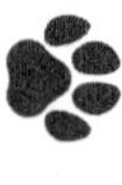
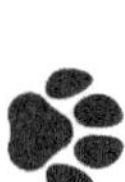
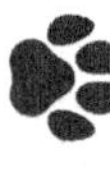
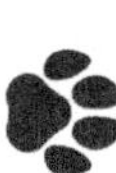
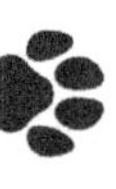
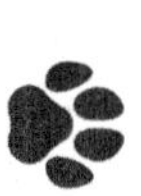
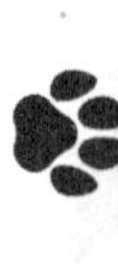

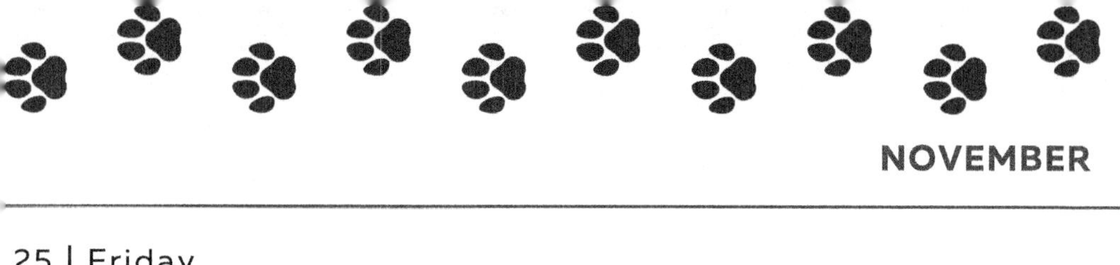

NOVEMBER

25 | Friday

26 | Saturday

27 | Sunday

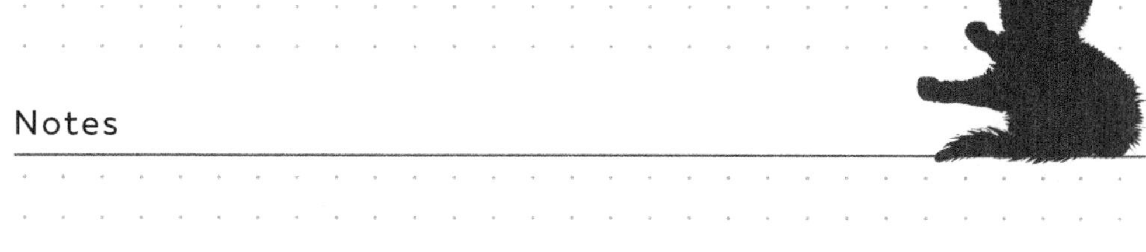

Notes

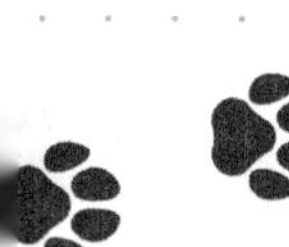
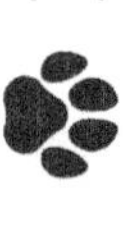

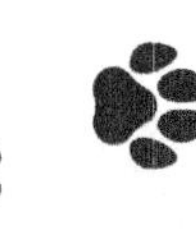
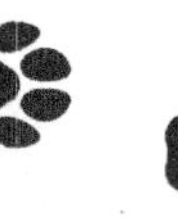

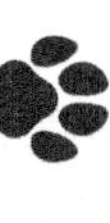
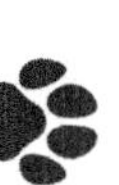
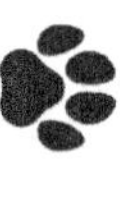
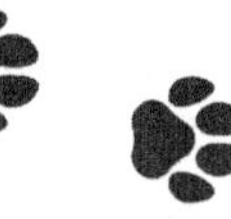
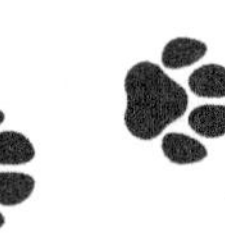

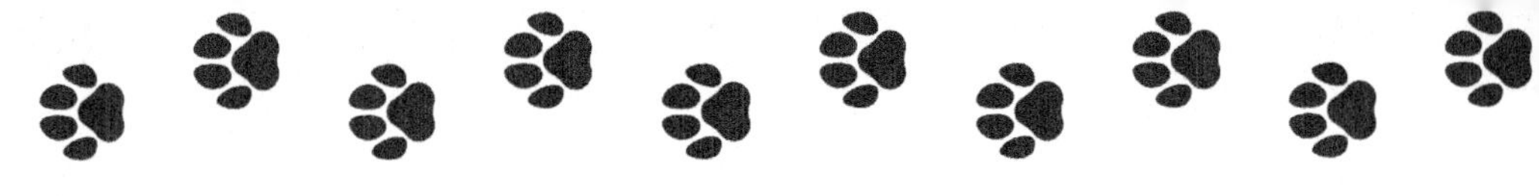

## DECEMBER

| Monday | Tuesday | Wednesday | Thursday |
|---|---|---|---|
| | | | 1 |
| 5 | 6 | 7 | 8 |
| 12 | 13 | 14 | 15 |
| 19 | 20 | 21 | 22 |
| 26 Boxing Day | 27 Substitute Bank Holiday for Christmas Day | 28 | 29 |

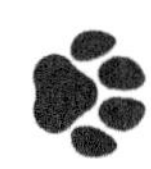 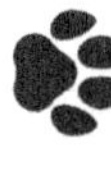 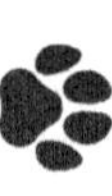 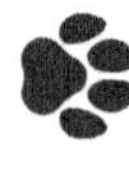 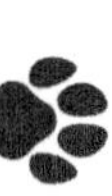 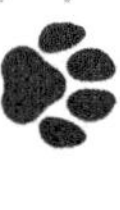 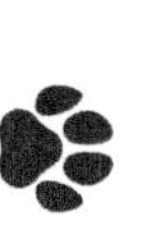 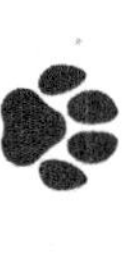 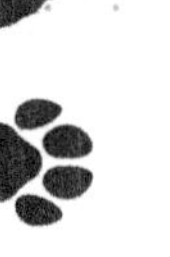

2022

| Friday | Saturday | Sunday |
|---|---|---|
| 2 | 3 | 4 |
| 9 | 10 | 11 |
| 16 | 17 | 18 |
| 23 | 24 Christmas Eve | 25 Christmas Day |
| 30 | 31 New Year's Eve | |

Goals

To Do

Reminder

Notes

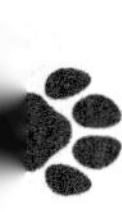
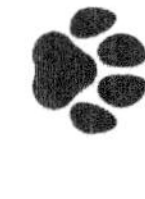
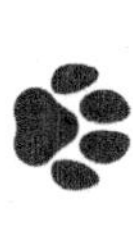
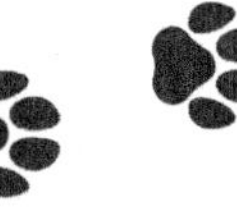
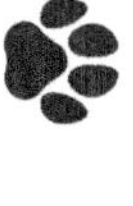
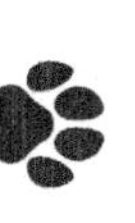

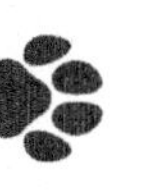

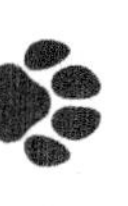
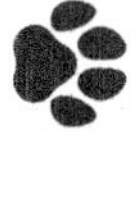

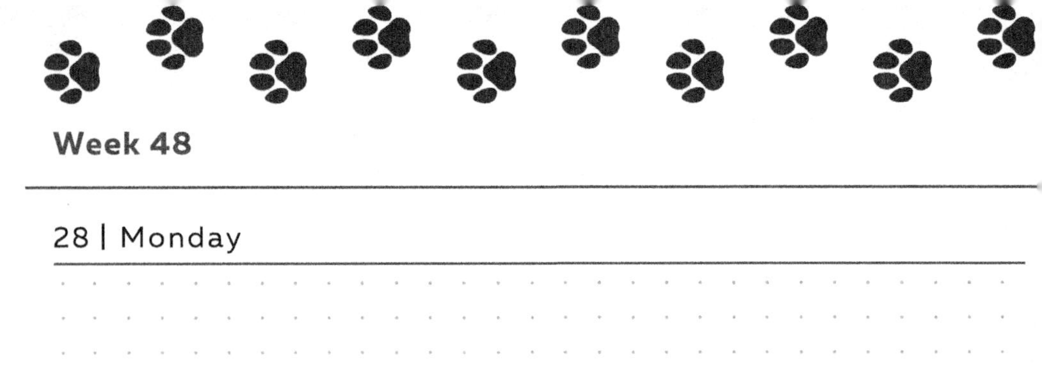

## Week 48

### 28 | Monday

### 29 | Tuesday

### 30 | Wednesday

### 1 | Thursday

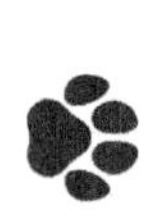 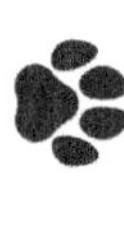 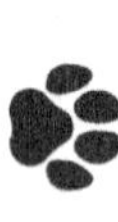 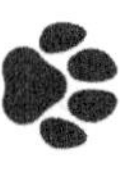 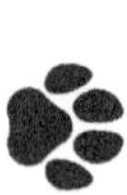 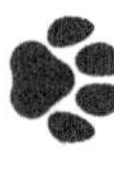 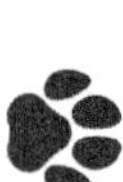 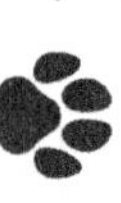  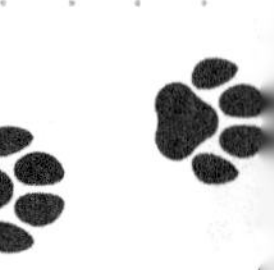

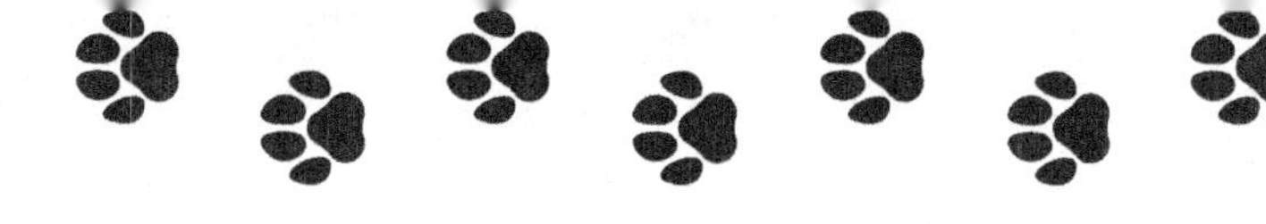



2 | Friday

3 | Saturday

4 | Sunday

Notes

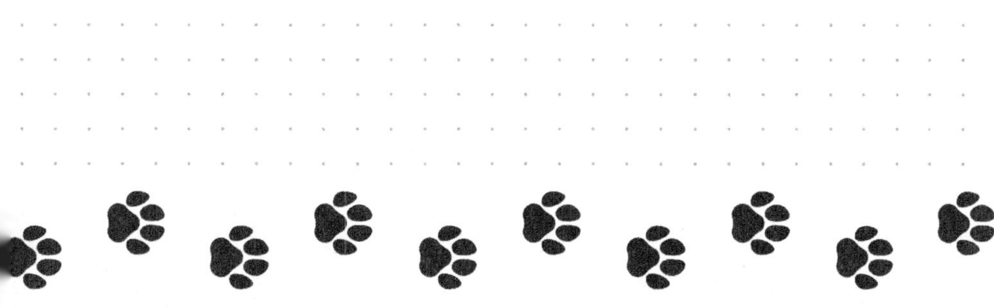

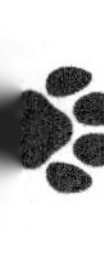

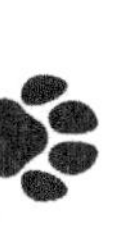

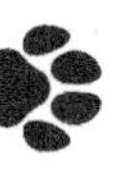

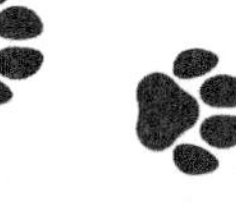

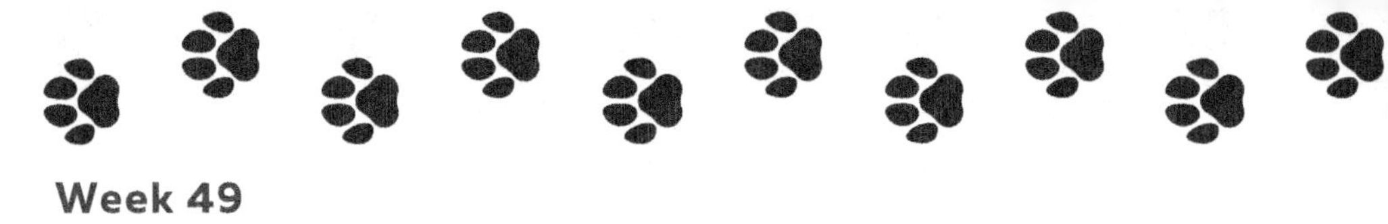

## Week 49

5 | Monday

6 | Tuesday

7 | Wednesday

8 | Thursday

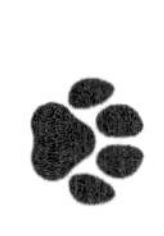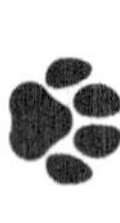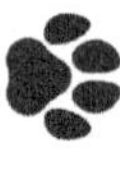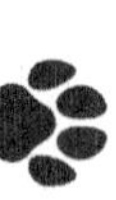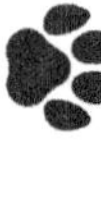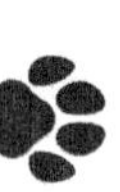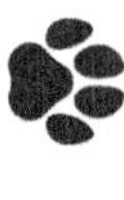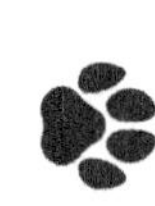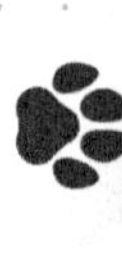

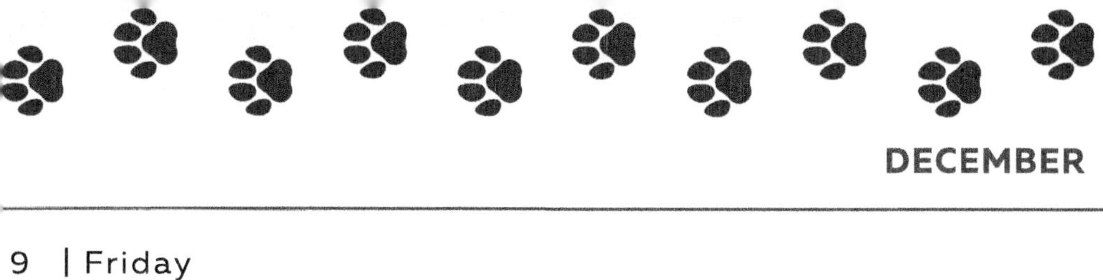

## DECEMBER

### 9 | Friday

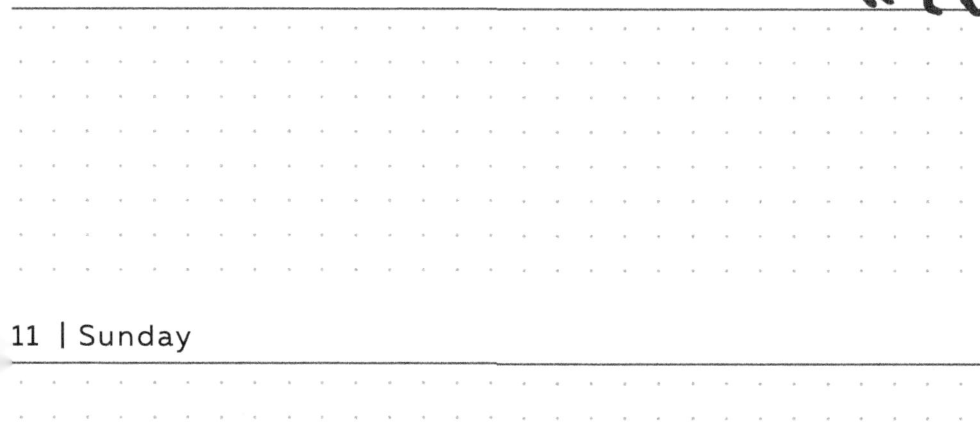

### 10 | Saturday

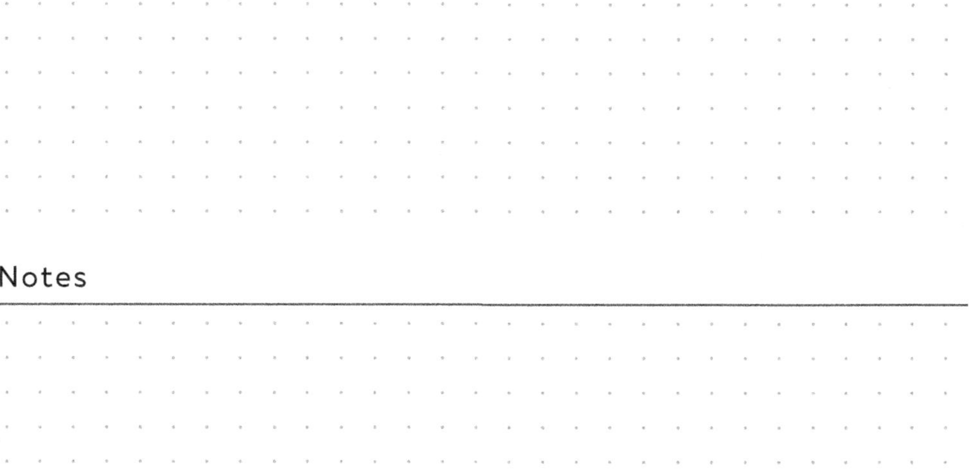

### 11 | Sunday

### Notes

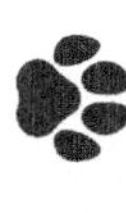
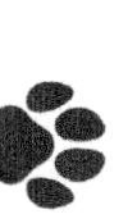
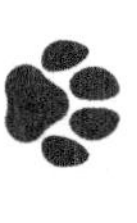
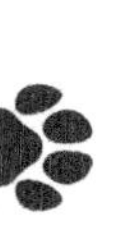
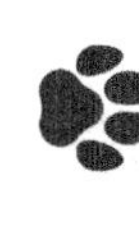
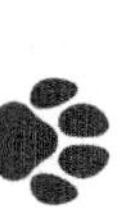
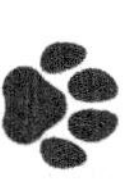
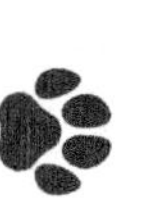
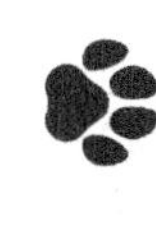

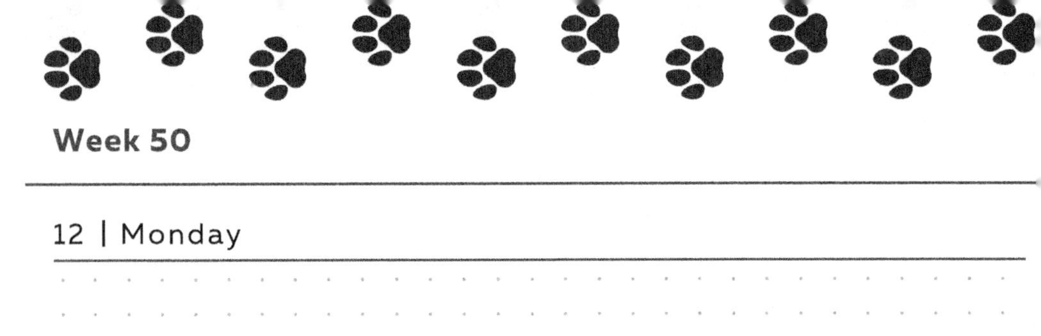

## Week 50

12 | Monday

13 | Tuesday

14 | Wednesday

15 | Thursday

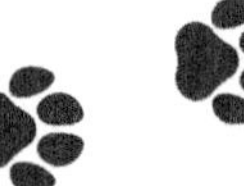
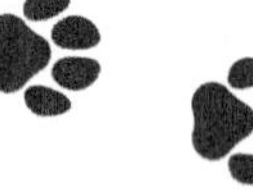
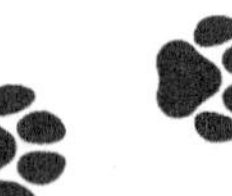
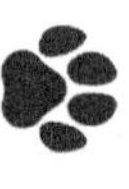
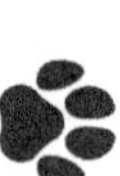
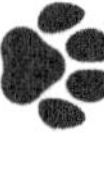
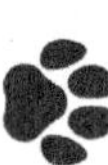
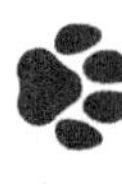
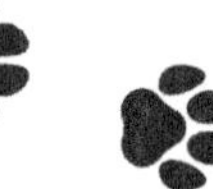
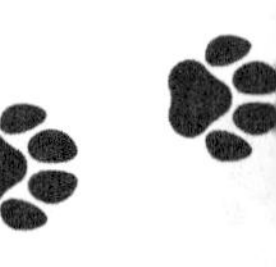

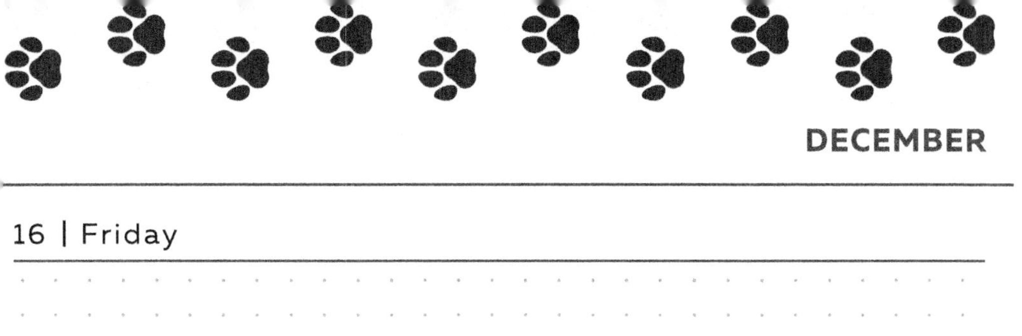

DECEMBER

16 | Friday

17 | Saturday

18 | Sunday

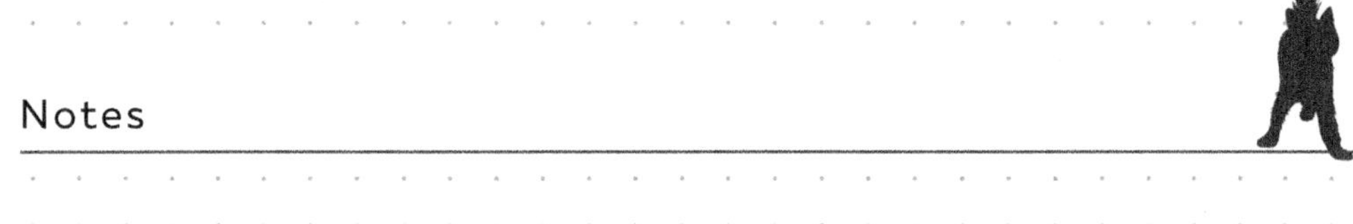

Notes

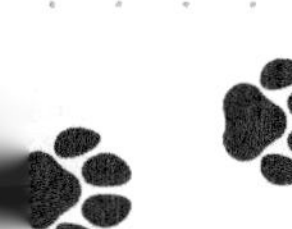
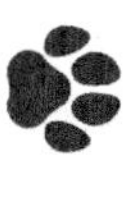
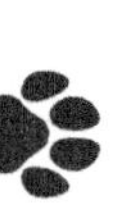
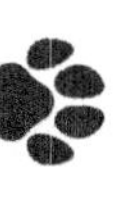
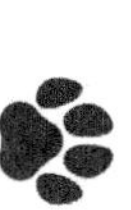
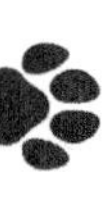
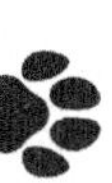
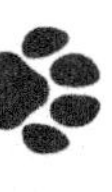
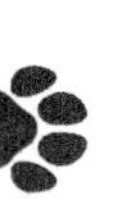
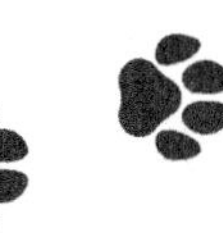

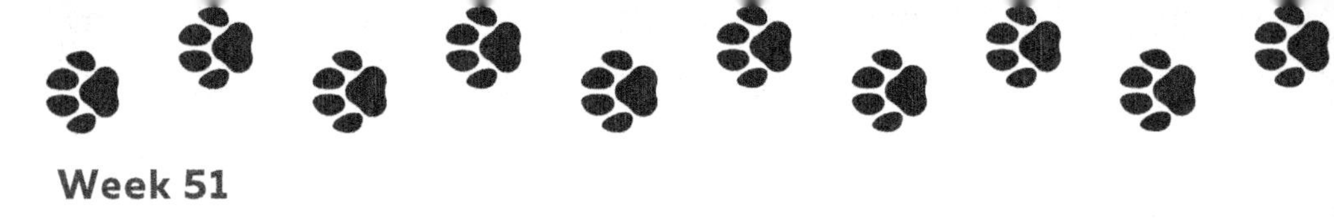

## Week 51

### 19 | Monday

### 20 | Tuesday

### 21 | Wednesday

### 22 | Thursday

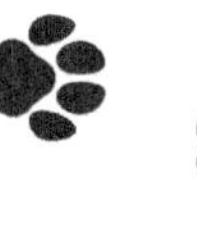
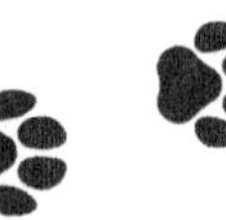
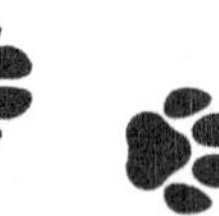
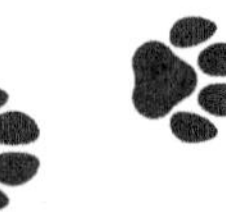
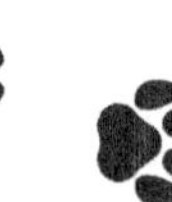
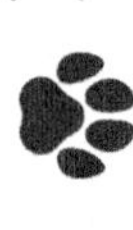
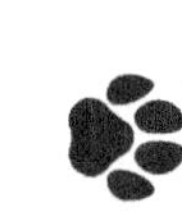
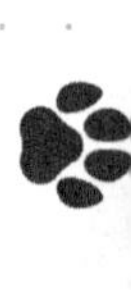

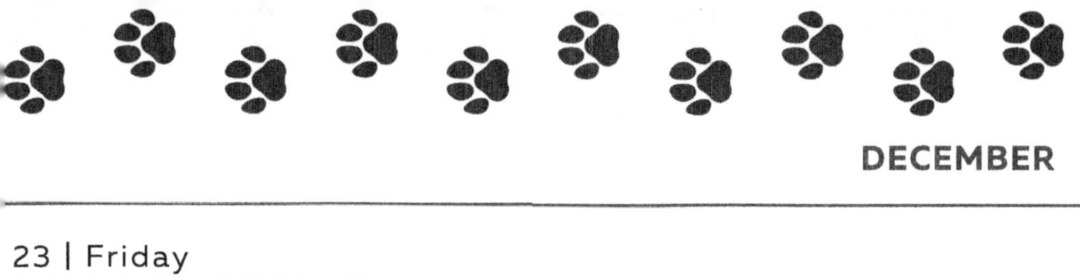

# DECEMBER

## 23 | Friday

## 24 | Saturday

Christmas Eve

## 25 | Sunday

Christmas Day

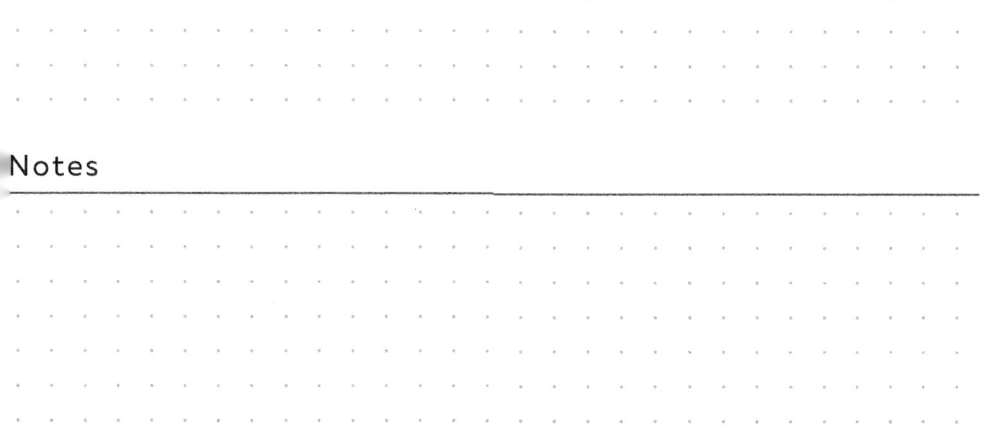

## Notes

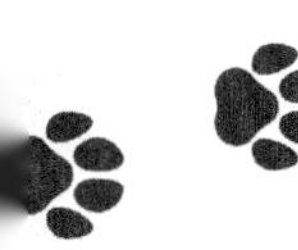
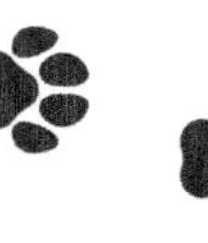
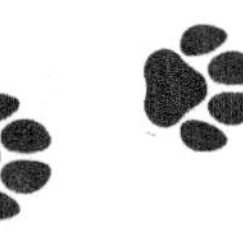
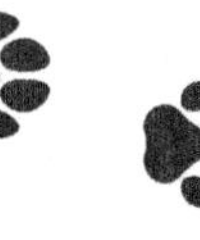
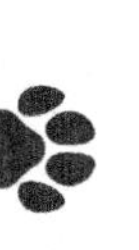

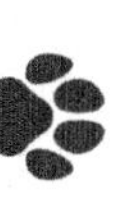
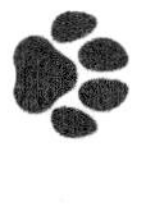
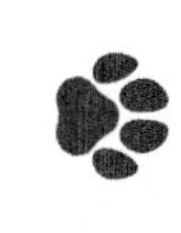

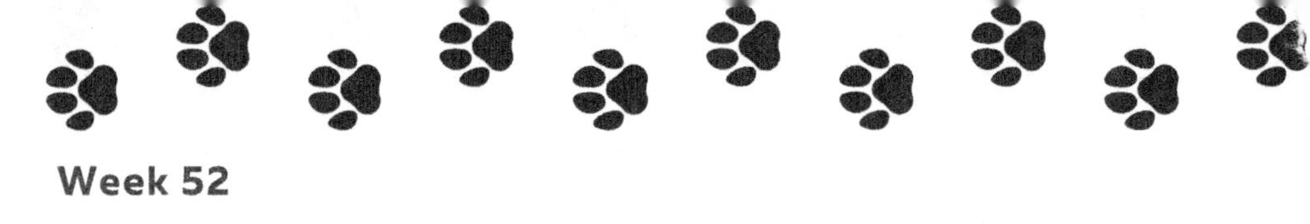

## Week 52

26 | Monday — Boxing Day

27 | Tuesday — Substitute Bank Holiday for Christmas Da

28 | Wednesday

29 | Thursday

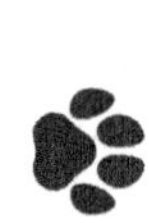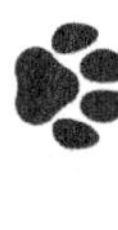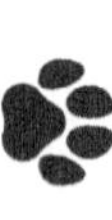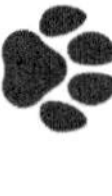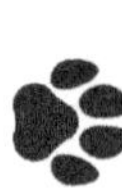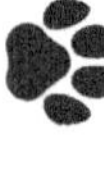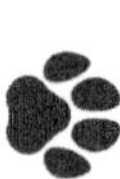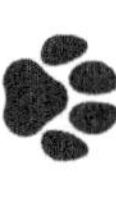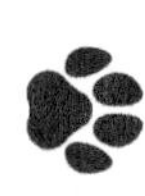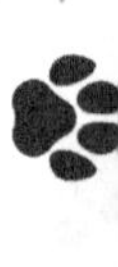

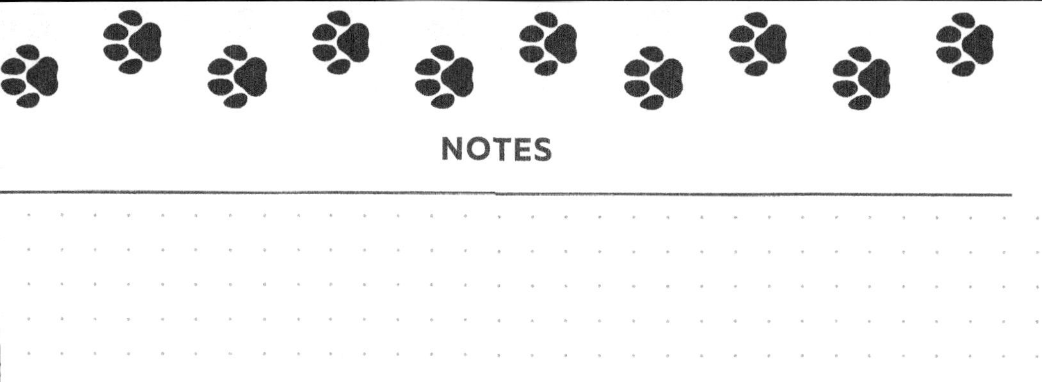

# NOTES

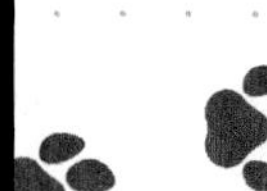

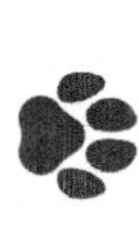
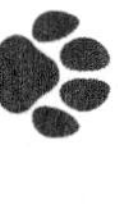
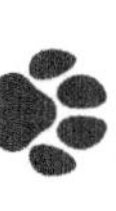
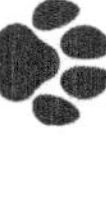
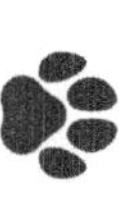
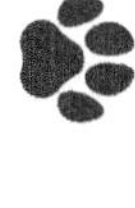
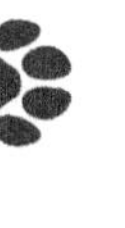

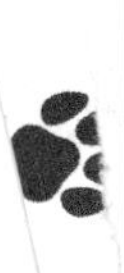

## NOTES

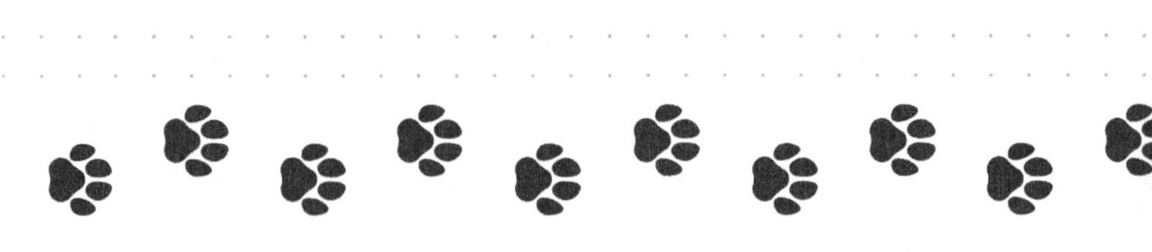

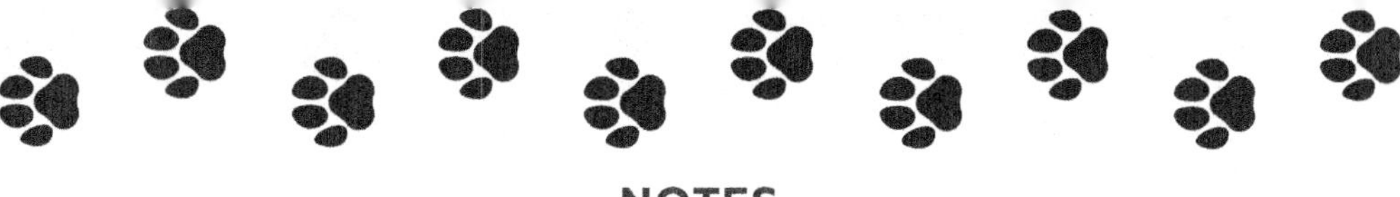

## NOTES

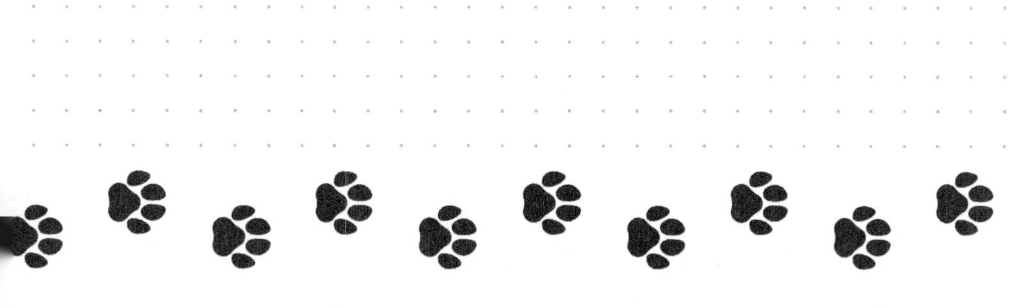

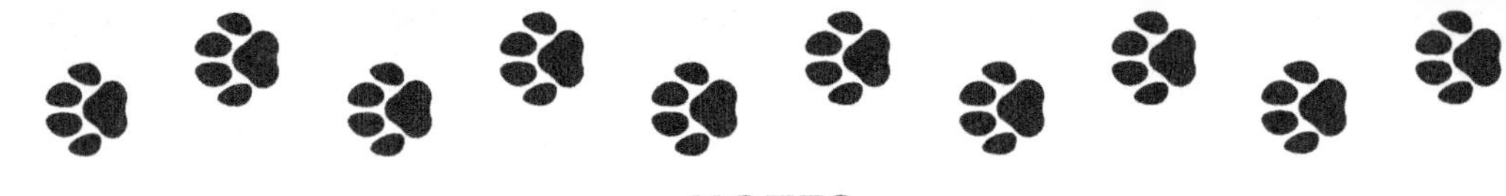

# NOTES

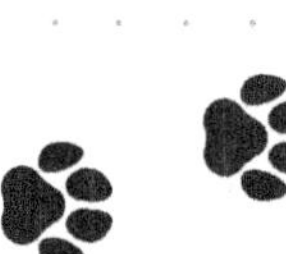
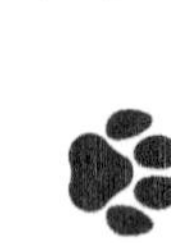
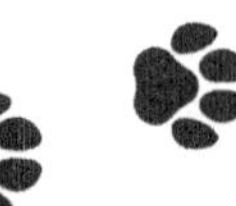
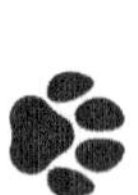
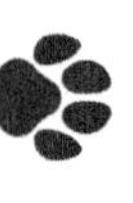
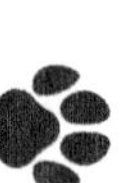
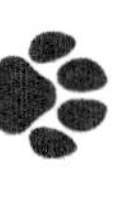
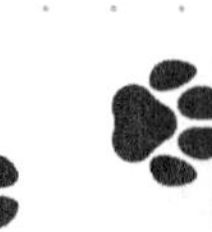

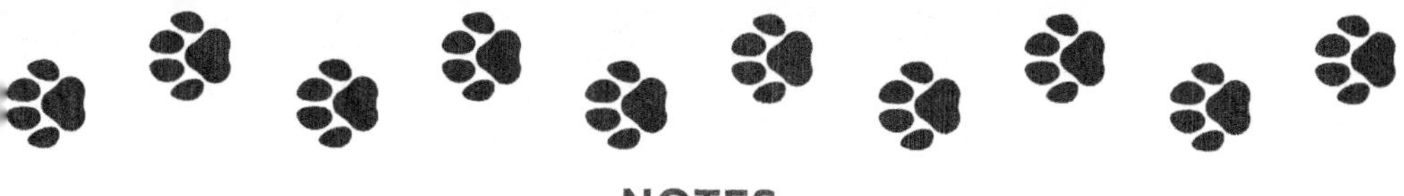

## NOTES

## NOTES

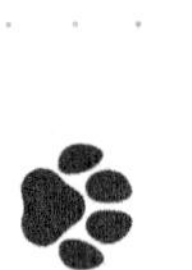
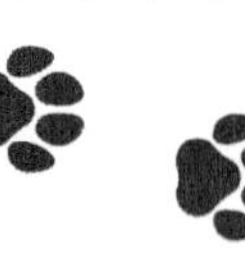
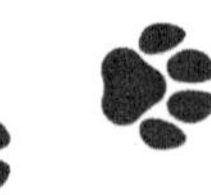
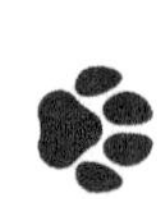
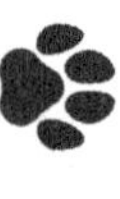
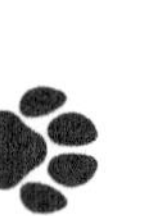

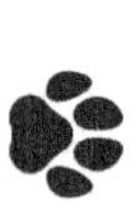
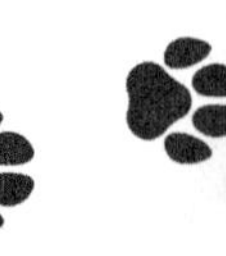

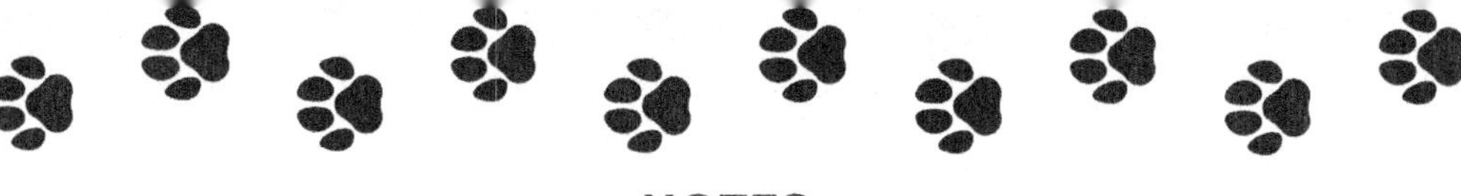

# NOTES

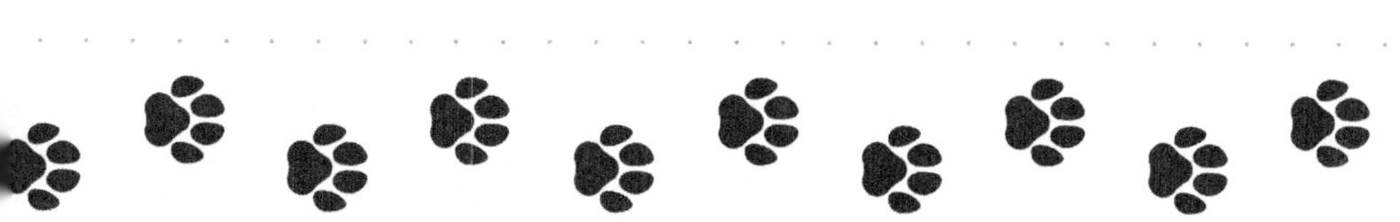
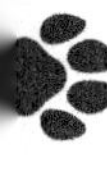
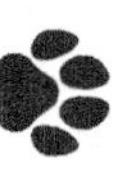
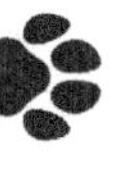
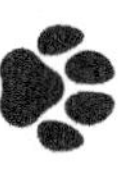
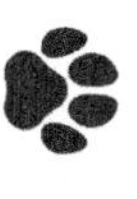
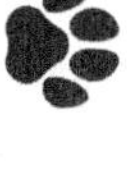

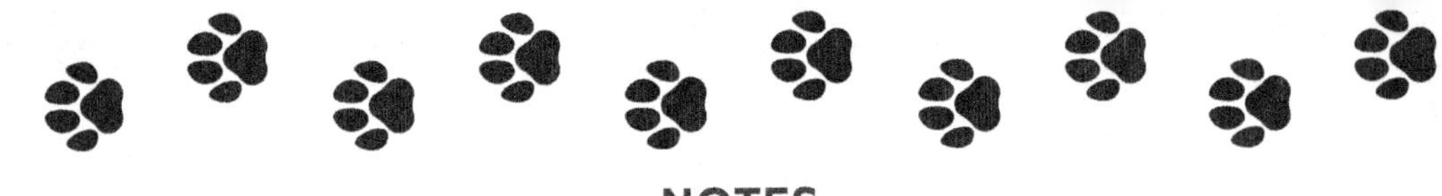

## NOTES

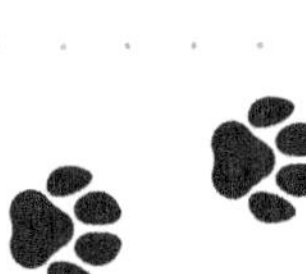
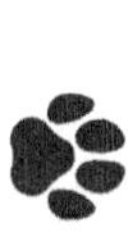
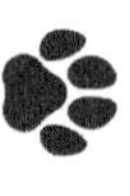
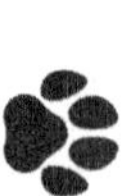

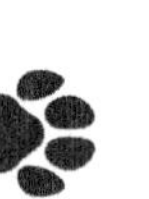
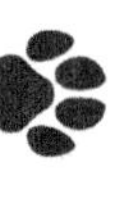
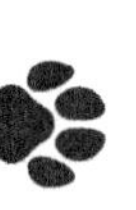

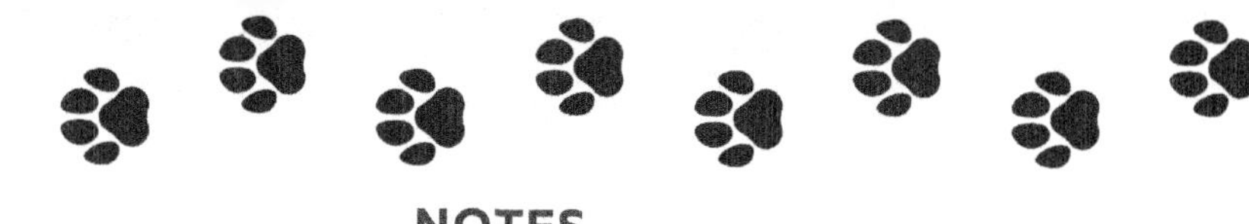

## NOTES

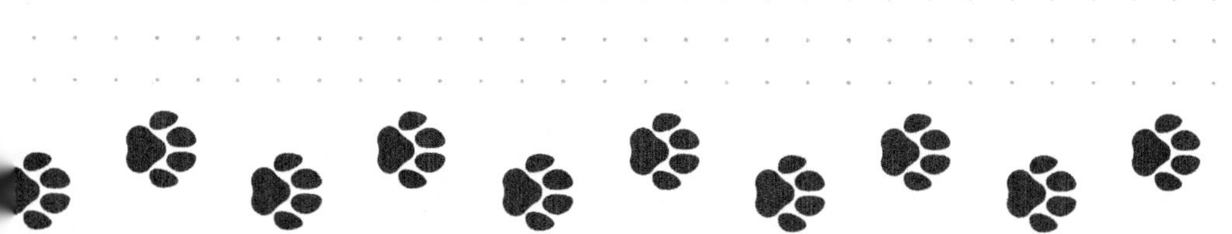

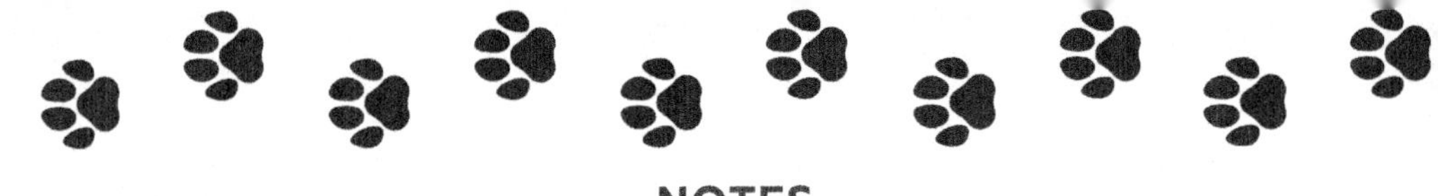

# NOTES

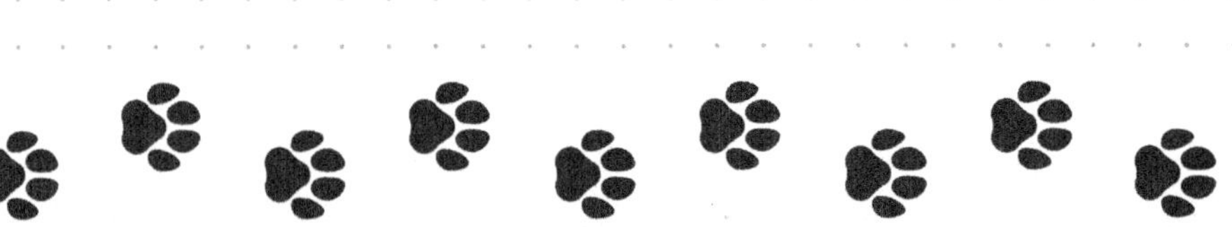

Printed in Great Britain
by Amazon